Walther and Houston's
Orthodontic Notes

Fifth edition

Edited and revised by

Malcolm L. Jones BDS (Wales), MSc (Lond), PhD (Wales), DOrth
RCS (Eng), FDS RCS (Edin)
Professor and Head of Dept. of Child Dental Health
University of Wales College of Medicine;
Honorary Consultant in Orthodontics to South Glamorgan and Gwent
Health Authorities

Richard G. Oliver BDS (Lond), MScD (Wales), LDS RCS (Eng),
FDS RCS (Edin)
Senior Lecturer in Orthodontics
University of Wales College of Medicine;
Honorary Consultant in Orthodontics to South Glamorgan Health
Authority

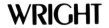

WRIGHT

Wright
An imprint of Butterworth-Heinemann Ltd
Linacre House, Jordan Hill, Oxford OX2 8DP

 A member of the Reed Elsevier plc group

OXFORD LONDON BOSTON
MUNICH NEW DELHI SINGAPORE SYDNEY
TOKYO TORONTO WELLINGTON

First edition, 1960
Reprinted, 1962
Reprinted, 1965
Second edition, 1967
Reprinted, 1972
Third edition, 1976
Reprinted, 1979
Fourth edition, 1983
Reprinted, 1985
Reprinted, 1990
Fifth edition, 1994

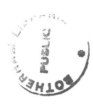

© Butterworth-Heinemann Ltd 1994

British Library Cataloguing in Publication Data
Walther, D.P.
  Walther and Houston's Orthodontic Notes.
  – 5Rev. ed
  I. Title II. Houston, W.J.B.
  III. Jones, Malcolm L. IV. Oliver,
  Richard G.
  617.463

ISBN 0 7236 1005 3

Composition by Scribe Design, Gillingham, Kent
Printed in Great Britain at the University Press, Cambridge

Contents

Contributors

Eli G. Absi   DDS, MScD, PhD, MSc Radiol
Senior Lecturer in Oral Radiology
University of Wales College of Medicine;
Consultant in Dental Surgery and Radiology to South
Glamorgan Health Authority

Radiology in Orthodontics – Chapter 17
Minor Oral Surgery in Relation to Orthodontics – Chapter 18

Adrian Sugar   BChD, FDS RCS
Consultant in Facio-Maxillary Surgery
The Maxillo-Facial Surgery Unit, Morriston Hospital, Swansea

The Role of Orthognathic Surgery – Chapter 19

Stephen Richmond   BDS, MScD, PhD, DOrth, FDS RCS
Reader in Dental Quality Assurance
University of Wales College of Medicine;
Honorary Consultant in Orthodontics to South Glamorgan
Health Authority.

Occlusal Indices – Chapter 22

Preface to the Fifth Edition

This book, first published in 1960, originally comprised the orthodontic notes taken from a series of lectures given to the undergraduate students at the Royal Dental Hospital, London, by Professor Walther. In the Preface to the first edition, Professor Walther stated that 'Orthodontic Notes' were published in the hope that they might be of some use to other students. He intended that they should form the basis around which both the undergraduate and postgraduate student might read and develop a knowledge of the subject. Little was Professor Walther to know how successful this format was to become and how widely this small text was to be read: indeed both of the current authors well remember referring to the second edition as undergraduates.

Following the early death of Professor Walther, Professor Houston was the natural successor to continue the updating and revision of the work, since he had been a Senior Lecturer at the Royal Dental Hospital and a contributor to the early editions. After the untimely and tragic loss of Bill Houston we were approached by the publishers to take over the mantle of revising this book for a further edition. We decided at a very early stage that since the text and style were very much Bill's, the new edition should be named 'Walther and Houston's Orthodontic Notes' and, with the agreement of Mrs. Houston, that a substantial portion of the royalties should be given to the prize established in his memory.

Bill Houston's Preface to the fourth edition is reprinted in full to remind readers of the continuing purpose of this work. Approaching the book afresh, as we have done, it is tempting to consider a revolutionary revision. However, over the years, based on a tried and tested formula, the text has been allowed to evolve. We would not wish to break with this tradition in the current edition; therefore the text is kept simple, brief and basic, avoiding detailed discussion wherever possible. The subject matter has been expanded in this edition to take account of the changes that have occurred in the speciality over the last decade. As in the past, long lists of references have been avoided: we would prefer to refer the reader to a companion and more exhaustive undergraduate text, *A Textbook of Orthodontics* by Houston, Stephens and Tulley and other similar texts.

Nevertheless, we hope that these notes will continue to provide a straightforward theoretical base on which the postgraduate, undergraduate or general dental practitioner may build knowledge as they develop an interest in the speciality of orthodontics.

M.L.J. and R.G.O.

Preface to the Fourth Edition

Since its first appearance in 1960, *Orthodontic Notes* has become a popular text with undergraduates. Although it has been reviewed extensively since that time, the intentions of Professor Walther have been followed: to present in a clear and concise fashion, the essentials of orthodontics required by undergraduate dental students and general dental practitioners. The brevity of presentation precludes detailed discussion of the many controversial topics in orthodontics. However, such debates are liable to be confusing rather than informative for the student who is being introduced to a subject. Thus a particular viewpoint is presented to hopefully provide a consistent and commonsense framework of ideas. This should provide an adequate theoretical basis for the undergraduate student or general dental practitioner, and should form a sound foundation for the student who wishes to go further to specialise in orthodontics.

W.J.B.H. 1983

Acknowledgements

There are several people who have contributed to the production of this book without whose cheerful co-operation the task would have been arduous if not impossible.

Lynne James has typed and retyped the manuscript, making sense of all sorts of scribbles and bizarre notation marks on early drafts. The Audio-visual Aids Department at the Dental School and Hospital in Cardiff has produced the bulk of the illustrations, and we are grateful to Mr Rodney Dollar for all his help and expertise. The illustrations for Chapter 19 were prepared by Bryce Cumisky of the Medical Illustration Department at St Lawrence Hospital in Chepstow, the original artwork provided by Peter Evans, Chief Maxillofacial Technologist.

We owe a debt of gratitude to Bill Houston and Norman Robertson, our respective teachers in the early stages of our orthodontic careers, for instilling into us an academic discipline of thought and deed, and leading by example. We are also grateful to the students, both undergraduate and postgraduate, whose searching questions keep us constantly thinking about what we are doing in orthodontics, and why.

Finally, but by no means least, we would like to acknowledge the help and support of our wives. Rhona Jones has helped with grammar, punctuation, and proofreading, while Sheila Oliver, being dentally qualified (and therefore as a potential reader of the book), has provided invaluable constructive comment.

Chapter 1

Introduction

Orthodontics has been defined as that branch of dental science concerned with genetic variation, development and growth of facial form. It is also concerned with the manner in which these factors affect the occlusion of the teeth and the function of associated organs. Thus, while orthodontic techniques are concerned with the treatment of irregularities of the teeth, the study of orthodontics as a whole includes the growth, development and function of the total orofacial complex.

The aims of orthodontic treatment have been suggested to be the production of improved occlusal function by the correction of irregularities and as a consequence the creation of better dental health and improved aesthetics. It would be envisaged that such an improvement in personal appearance might later contribute to greater mental and physical well-being on the part of the individual patient. Although there might be some dispute as to whether all of these aims are routinely achievable in all patients, it is an important concept to grasp at the outset that no orthodontic treatment should harm the patient. Such harm might occur by making the tooth arrangement or facial profile worse or could involve leaving unsightly residual gaps after the inappropriate extraction of teeth. It is important that each treatment and thus each appliance approach should be matched to the individual. Similarly, the appropriate level of professional skill should also be matched to the presenting problem. This will mean that while some patients may be treated by simple means in the general dental practice environment, many others will require referral to a specialist practitioner with training in more advanced techniques.

The general dental practitioner attends to the dental well-being of the patient. This would include both the monitoring and management of the developing occlusion. They should have sufficient orthodontic knowledge to enable them to know when they might intervene to improve tooth arrangement, but also when it is best to refer for either an expert opinion or a more complex treatment.

1

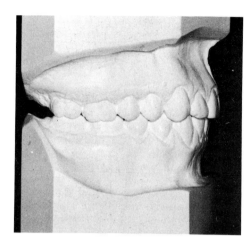

Figure 1.1 Normal occlusion of the permanent teeth

Ideal occlusion is a hypothetical concept based on the anatomy of the teeth. It is rarely, if ever, found in nature. However, it provides a standard by which all other occlusions may be judged.

Normal occlusion (Figure 1.1) is commonly described as 'An occlusion within the accepted deviation of the ideal'. This vague definition means that there are no clear limits to the range of normal occlusion. However, in general, minor variations in the alignment of the teeth which are not of aesthetic or functional importance might be considered as being consistent with a normal occlusion. Edward Angle, who is credited with the modern development of orthodontics as a speciality, provided the first clear definition of normal occlusion. He related it to the arrangement of the occlusal contact of the first permanent molars, the mesio buccal cusp of the maxillary first permanent molar occluding with the buccal groove of the opposing mandibular first permanent molar. He suggested that if such a relationship existed and the teeth were arranged in a smoothly curving line of occlusion then a normal occlusion would be the result.

Malocclusion is an irregularity in the occlusion beyond the accepted range of normal. The fact that an individual has a malocclusion is not in itself a justification for treatment. Only if is it possible to say with certainty that the patient will benefit aesthetically or functionally and only if they are suitable and willing to undergo treatment should orthodontic intervention be considered.

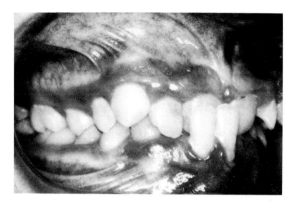

Figure 1.2 A traumatic occlusion. Note the gingival recession on the lower central incisors

The scope and aims of orthodontic treatment

- The improvement of facial and dental aesthetics.
- The alignment of the teeth to eliminate stagnation areas.
- The elimination of premature contacts which give rise to mandibular displacements and may contribute to later muscle or joint pain.
- The elimination of traumatic irregularities of the teeth (Figure 1.2).
- The alignment of prominent teeth which are liable to be damaged.
- The alignment of irregular teeth prior to bridgework, crowns or partial dentures.
- The alignment of periodontally involved teeth prior to splinting.
- The alignment and planned positioning of teeth in the jaws prior to orthognathic surgery.
- To assist the eruption and alignment of displaced teeth.

Orthodontic treatment options

There are seven basic treatment approaches to the management and correction of malocclusion:

1. *No treatment.* This involves the acceptance of mild irregularity on the principle that limited crowding will often be far better than any residual post-treatment extraction space.

Limited resources should be concentrated on patients with more severe malocclusions.

2. *Extraction only.* To be considered only where the degree and position of crowding is favourable, as are the local tooth angulations. Extraction of teeth will allow spontaneous movement and may provide an acceptable result in a limited number of cases.

3. *Removable appliance treatment.* Where tooth position, inclination and angulations are favourable, a removable appliance may correct a malocclusion by simple tipping movements about the apical third of the root (see Chapter 14). Removable appliances are most efficient and are best tolerated in the upper dental arch.

4. *Single arch fixed appliances.* These may be used where there are limited treatment aims, usually involving corrections of either rotations or angulations of teeth. They may on occasions be used in the lower arch for the purposes of alignment or for space closure where bodily movement is necessary. In this situation it may be used in conjunction with an upper removable appliance.

5. *Full upper and lower arch fixed appliances.* These appliances are attached to most of the maxillary and mandibular teeth and allow full correction of all teeth in three planes of space (see Chapter 15).

6. *Functional appliances.* These specialized removable appliances consist of an upper and lower segment which are fixed together such as to hold the mandibular dental arch in a postured position. They are most appropriately employed in those patients with retrusive mandibular teeth and jaw. These appliances appear to be most effective in patients where there is current active growth (see Chapter 16).

7. *Orthognathic surgery.* This is a complex treatment approach involving a combination of both fixed appliances and surgery to the jaws. By such means large discrepancies of the jaws may be corrected in suitable patients when growth has largely ceased (see Chapter 19). Careful planning together with the timing of surgery demand early and expert inter-speciality appraisal.

The timing of orthodontic treatment

The deciduous dentition
Treatment at this stage is hardly ever indicated. Examples of possible exceptions are where a malpositioned tooth may give rise

to marked mandibular displacement, or where a supernumerary tooth is creating a localized problem. It will be important, however, to identify and make an early referral for those patients where significant jaw discrepancy or facial asymmetry are apparent during these early stages of growth.

The early mixed dentition
The planned extraction of extensively carious first permanent molars, balancing extractions of deciduous teeth and serial extractions may be undertaken during this stage (see Chapter 6). Space maintainers may be fitted and simple orthodontic treatment to correct an instanding incisor or alternatively to eliminate a mandibular displacement may be indicated (see Chapter 8). Only treatment which can be completed rapidly and which will be stable should be attempted. Prolonged appliance wear at this stage is to be avoided and is unlikely in any event to be longer than between 3 and 6 months. The types of treatment that are employed in the early mixed dentition are intended to either eliminate or at a minimum reduce the severity of a developing malocclusion.

The late mixed and early permanent dentition
At this stage, the greater part of orthodontic treatment is carried out. Most of the permanent teeth have erupted and there is little further growth in arch width, thus crowding can be reliably estimated. In the majority of children the jaw relationship changes only to a limited extent after the age of 10 years (see Chapter 2) and so it is possible to plan and carry out orthodontic treatment with the confidence that major growth changes are not likely to affect the treatment adversely. It is at this stage that most definitive active treatment to correct malocclusion will be performed and it has been suggested that children in this age group are often more willing to wear appliances than are older adolescents and adults.

The late permanent dentition
It is important to recognize that orthodontic treatment may be undertaken at any age. In North America and Western Europe, a rapidly increasing number of treatments are being undertaken for the adult patient. However, treatment planning and mechanics will usually require modification from that which is appropriate in the growing child (see Chapter 20).

Chapter 2

The facial skeleton

Growth of the face and skull

The bones of the cranial vault develop in the membranes covering the brain in the embryo. Centres of ossification appear and the bones expand so that by birth they are related to one another at sutures, although some areas – the fontanelles, still have a membranous covering (Figure 2.1). The sutures are sites at which limited movement of the bones is possible and where growth in the size of the cranial vault can occur. They are fibrous joints with little inherent growth potential: growth at the sutures occurs by their expansion due to growth in volume of the cranial contents. In addition to the increase in surface area, the bones of the cranial vault are thickened as a result of periosteal apposition. They consist of outer and inner tables of compact bone separated by a layer of cancellous bone. Where functional demands require, for example at muscle attachments and sites of stress concentration, the outer table may be elevated into ridges and crests. This happens at the temporal and nuchal crests and at the supra-orbital ridges where the space between the inner and outer tables becomes pneumatized.

The cranial base comprises the bones that develop from the cartilaginous chondrocranium of the embryo. At birth, cartilage remains at sites where growth can occur: the synchondroses. These have a structure that resembles that of the epiphyseal cartilages of the long bones, except that in this instance growth occurs in both of the bones contributing to the joint. The spheno-ethmoidal and spheno-occipital synchondroses are responsible for growth in length of the cranial base. The former fuses at about 6 years of age after which there is little growth change at the midline in the floor of the anterior cranial fossa. This relatively stable area of the anterior cranial base is used as a reference structure from which growth changes elsewhere in the facial skeleton can be measured. The upper facial skeleton is related to the anterior cranial fossa, while the mandible is related to the middle

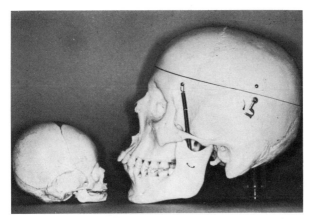

a

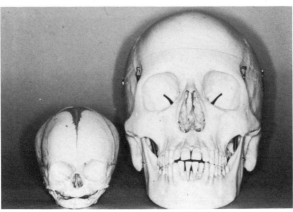

b

Figure 2.1 Neonate and adult skulls. Note the difference in proportions between the facial skeleton and the calvarium at the different ages. The proportions of the facial skeleton also change with age

cranial fossa at its articulation with the temporal bone (Figure 2.2). The length of the cranial base thus has an influence on jaw relationships, and growth at the spheno-occipital synchondrosis, which continues until about the age of puberty, has an influence on relative jaw position. Growth of the cranial base is not influenced by orthodontic means and is probably under fairly tight genetic control.

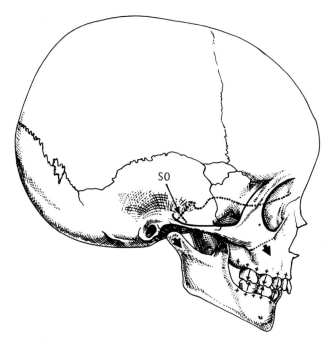

Figure 2.2 The maxilla grows downwards and forwards in part due to growth at sutures (i.e. displacement) and in part by surface apposition and remodelling of bone (i.e. drift). The mandible grows downwards and forwards from its cranial articulations at a greater rate than does the maxilla. Thus the intermaxillary space grows in height and is bridged by vertical growth at the alveolar processes and eruption of the teeth. The midline cranial base is indicated by a dotted line. Growth at the spheno-occipital synchondrosis (SO) increases the distance between the cranial articulations of the maxilla and mandible

The facial skeleton

The maxilla grows downwards and forwards from the anterior cranial base, in part as a result of growth at the circum-maxillary suture system and in part as a result of extensive surface apposition and remodelling of bone. In general terms the outward and downward facing surfaces of the maxilla are formative, in particular at the alveolar process and on the oral surface of the palate, with corresponding resorption on the nasal surfaces. Thus the maxilla grows downwards and forwards in part due to drift (surface remodelling). The sutures of the upper facial skeleton are structurally comparable with those of the cranial vault and, like them, probably have little independent growth potential. However, it has not been possible to isolate the primary growth-promoting forces in the upper facial skeleton. Growth of the nasal septum and of the eyeballs have been cited as possible factors. Probably no single factor controls and directs growth of the upper facial skeleton. It has been shown that heavy forces applied to the maxillary teeth by orthodontic appliances can, according to the direction of traction, reduce or accelerate growth at the maxillary sutures. However, this is of limited practical application because, following such treatment, the natural growth pattern tends to reassert itself and there is a corresponding catch-up or lag so that the ultimate facial pattern is little affected. Only if such treatment were continued for many years until facial growth was nearly complete would lasting appreciable changes be achieved.

Growth in the overall length of the mandible takes place largely at the condyle, but of course comparable remodelling periosteal growth changes take place to maintain the form of the mandible. It is a question of continuing controversy whether growth at the condyles propels the mandible downwards and forwards from the glenoid fossa or whether condylar growth is merely adaptive to other factors that carry the mandible downwards and forwards. It seems probable that the condylar cartilage has an appreciable inherent growth potential but that it can be affected by local factors. However, its growth can be influenced only to a very limited extent by orthodontic appliance treatment. Proponents of functional appliances (see Chapter 16) claim that condylar growth can be controlled but this is still a matter of debate. The practitioner is wise to plan treatment on the assumption that his appliances will not influence condylar growth.

The mandible grows downwards and forwards from its articulation with the middle cranial fossa faster than does the maxilla (Figure 2.2). Anteroposteriorly this is largely compensated for by the growth of the spheno-occipital synchondrosis which carries the maxilla forward. However, the tendency is for mandibular prognathism (i.e. projection from under the cranial structures) to increase slightly faster than does maxillary prognathism.

Vertically, the distance between the mandibular and maxillary bases, the intermaxillary space, increases in height. This is bridged by vertical growth of the teeth and alveolar processes which adapt to changes in height and shape of the intermaxillary space. The vertical relationship of the mandible to the upper facial structures is determined not only by growth at the condyles, but by the lengths of the muscles and fascia attached to it: principally the muscles of mastication which pass between the mandible and the

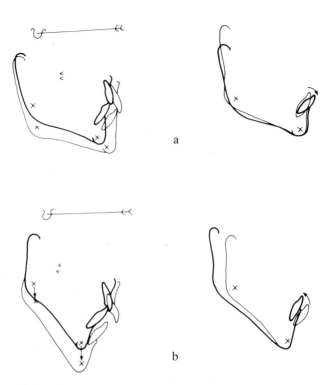

Figure 2.3 Mandibular growth rotations: a, anterior (closing) growth rotation; b, posterior (opening) growth rotation. The crosses indicate hypothetical stable points in the mandible, purely for the purposes of illustration. Where the posterior and anterior facial heights grow by different amounts, a mandibular growth rotation will occur but will to a large extent be masked by remodelling at the lower and posterior borders of the mandible. This is revealed when mandibular outlines are superimposed on the stable structures. The relative orientation of the lower incisors within the face is usually maintained by dento-alveolar adaptation. In most children, growth rotations are small

rest of the craniofacial skeleton and the suprahyoid muscles below. Growth in length of these is in turn influenced by growth in length of the neck and the cervical vertebrae. Many other factors, such as the physiological need to maintain an airway, play a part in determining mandibular positions.

This means that superimposed on the downward and forward translation of the mandible relative to the cranial base, there may be minor degrees of anterior or posterior rotation (Figure 2.3) depending on the balance of growth between the condyle and the muscles attached to the mandible. As discussed below, the position of the teeth and alveolar structures adapts to these changes in mandibular relationships.

Patterns of growth

At birth, the volume of the brain case is greater than that of the face (Figure 2.1), but after the age of 6 years there is little further growth in volume because the brain has nearly reached its adult size. The facial skeleton grows steadily over a much longer period and thus in the adult forms a much larger proportion of the skull than in the child and projects further forward from under the brain case (Figure 2.1). The infant's face is relatively broad, but with postnatal growth the proportions of the face change, growth in breadth being least and in depth most. Thus on average the face in an adult appears longer and narrower and projects further forward than in the child. Some of the most noticeable changes in facial characteristics are due to the fact that the eyes are relatively large in the infant but, like the brain, grow relatively little after the age of 6 years while the nose is very much more prominent in the adult than in the child. These changes do not affect the occlusion, but changes in the character of the face obviously affect the appearance of the dentition in the face: even with a normal occlusion, the teeth of the 9-year-old child may seem to be rather large and prominent but with growth of the rest of the face and in particular of the nose, the impression changes.

Growth spurts and kinetics

The different tissues of the body grow at different rates, forming a variety of curves when the tissue size is plotted against time. Growth of the skeleton follows the general somatic growth pattern: there is an initial acceleration after birth; this then slows until there is another growth spurt between 6 and 7 years of age. This acceleration may last for only 3–4 months and usually comes earlier in girls than boys. However, the spurt of most interest to orthodontists is the prepubertal acceleration. This again lasts a few months, occurring (on average) at 12 years in girls and 14 years in boys. There is a large variation in the timing (standard deviation is 1 year), and it may occur as late as 16 years of age in boys.

During this prepubertal period of rapid somatic growth there is some evidence that teeth move more rapidly in response to forces. In particular, certain appliance techniques are more effective:

examples would be functional appliances (see Chapter 16) and extra-oral traction (see Chapter 15). For this reason, attempts have been made to try to predict growth spurts in children so that treatment may be prescribed to coincide with these periods – such predictive techniques have so far proved to be unreliable.

It is also of some interest to clinicians to know when the majority of facial growth has ceased. This can affect the treatment planning (see Chapter 20) but is particularly important in the timing of orthognathic surgery (see Chapter 19). For the purposes of treatment planning, the majority of facial growth is usually complete by 16–17 years of age. Even so, there is now some evidence that small increments of growth to the face occur into middle age; however, this unlikely to be of any significance in the treatment of malocclusion.

Facial growth and the occlusion

The alveolar bone is highly adaptable, depending for its presence and location on the presence and position of the teeth: remove a tooth and the associated alveolar process resorbs; move a tooth and it remodels.

Dento-alveolar compensation

Because the upper and lower teeth erupt into the common zone between lips, cheeks and tongue, they tend to be guided towards one another to establish an occlusion and to compensate for any transverse or anteroposterior malrelationships of the jaws. Variations in vertical jaw relationships are compensated to a greater or lesser degree by eruption of the teeth and growth of the alveolar processes. Where the skeletal malrelationships are too severe, the dento-alveolar compensation described above may not be sufficient to establish a normal occlusion and so crossbite, open bite and anteroposterior arch malrelationships may develop. However, arch malrelationships will often be less severe than might have been expected from the jaw malrelationship (Figure 2.4c). In some cases dento-alveolar compensation does not operate because of variations in soft-tissue patterns. For example, if the upper lip is short and the lips are habitually parted the upper incisors will tend to be proclined and are not guided towards the lower incisors. The lower incisors will then continue to erupt, possibly until they contact the palate. Dento-alveolar compensation is not always advantageous: in some cases of mandibular retrusion, for example, compensation occurs by

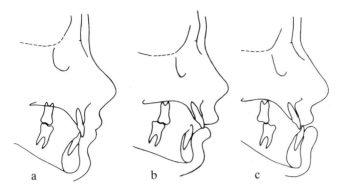

Figure 2.4 Skeletal patterns: a, Class I; b, Class II; c, Class III

retroclination of the upper incisors (see Figure 11.1). This type of incisor relationship is usually associated with a deep overbite and may be traumatic as well as being unsightly.

Dento-alveolar adaptation

As the face grows, the intermaxillary space increases in height and anteroposterior jaw relationships may change. As a result of vertical growth of the teeth and alveolar processes, occlusal contacts and the soft-tissue environment of the teeth, the existing occlusion or malocclusion tends to be maintained. Dento-alveolar adaptation is a dynamic process, while dento-alveolar compensation refers to an existing state of affairs: on examining a patient, it is possible to ascertain to what extent dento-alveolar compensation exists. Only with records obtained on more than one occasion can one identify the nature and amount of dento-alveolar adaptation that may have occurred over that time period.

Dento-alveolar adaptation is greatest vertically, in response to vertical growth of the intermaxillary space. Little change in transverse jaw relationships occurs with growth. Where changes in anteroposterior jaw relationships occur there will usually be corresponding dento-alveolar adaptation. Most commonly, the mandible grows forwards slightly more than the maxilla and the upper incisors procline while the lower incisors retrocline. The proclination of the upper incisors does not produce spacing because the upper buccal segments come forward by a comparable amount. Retroclination of the lower incisors usually results in crowding. If the adaptive mechanisms cannot cope with the extent of the change in jaw relationships there will be occlusal change. This most often happens where there is a Class III arch relationship (Figure 2.4c) and there is little or no incisor overbite. Growth rotations of the mandible may be superimposed upon the changes described above. Such growth rotations initiate dento-alveolar adaptation which may in turn lead to lower incisor crowding. With a posterior growth rotation (Figure 2.3b) the lower incisors tend to become retroclined under the influence of the soft-tissue integument of the face so that their relationship to upper facial reference planes changes little. The buccal segments do not move back by a corresponding amount and so lower arch crowding may appear or become more severe.

Anterior mandibular growth rotations (Figure 2.3a) are associated with proclination of the lower incisors within the alveolar process and with an upward and forward path of eruption of the buccal teeth. Measured to a reference plane in the upper face, the lower incisors do not become proclined but maintain their inclination. Provided that the forward movement of anterior and posterior teeth are in balance there should be no change in the space conditions of the lower arch. However, the lower incisors, through contact with the upper incisors, are often prevented from adapting completely, particularly if at the same time the mandible is growing forwards to a greater extent than is the maxilla. In these circumstances the lower buccal teeth will encroach on space for the lower labial segment with the development of lower incisor crowding.

Orthodontic treatment planning for the child is based on the hypothesis that the growth changes which take place will be within the normal range and so will have only minor effects on the occlusion. This is satisfactory for the majority of patients but occasionally unforeseen changes may occur and treatment planning will have to be revised. Many attempts have been made to predict accurately the future growth trends of the facial skeleton in the individual, but at the present time this is not possible.

The skeletal relationship

The relationship between the jaws has important effects on dental arch relationship. Unless lateral skull radiographs are available (see Figure 2.6), jaw relationship is assessed from the clinical examination of the patient. Skeletal relationships should be considered in three axes: anteroposterior, vertical and transverse.

Clinical assessment

Anteroposterior
This sagittal relationship between the jaws (the skeletal pattern) depends on the length of maxilla, length of mandible and the length of the cranial base between its articulation with the maxilla and the temporomandibular joint. The skeletal pattern is assessed by examining the profile as the patient sits unsupported, with the head in the free postural position and the mandible in the rest position or with the teeth in centric occlusion (the mandible must not be postured or displaced). When the mandible is normally related to the maxilla, the skeletal pattern is Class I; when it is posteriorly positioned relative to the maxilla, the skeletal pattern is Class II; and when it is too far forward the skeletal pattern is Class III (Figure 2.4). Subjective assessment of this sort is open to error and if there is a marked discrepancy between the thickness of the upper and lower lips, or a prominent chin 'button' (pogonion), the soft-tissue profile may give a misleading impression of the skeletal pattern. Nevertheless, this method of assessment is usually more accurate than attempts to judge skeletal relationships with the lips retracted. Minor variations in skeletal pattern are of little clinical importance and the larger variations from normal, which do have a bearing on aetiology and treatment, can readily be recognized.

Vertical
The space between the upper and lower skeletal bases is the intermaxillary space. The height of this space depends on the shape of the mandible and on the resting lengths of the muscles of mastication. Where the anterior height of the intermaxillary space is large an open bite may be found (see Chapter 8).

The angle between Frankfort and mandibular planes (see Figure 2.7) gives an index of anterior intermaxillary height. The average value for this angle is 27°, with a normal range of 5° in either direction. If the Frankfort mandibular planes angle is large the anterior intermaxillary height will usually be increased. It is not easy to estimate by eye the size of the Frankfort mandibular planes angle. Various forms of protractor are available, but it is perhaps simpler to compare the lower (Menton-Ans) and middle (Ans-Glabella) facial heights (Figure 2.7 and see Appendix II). In the well-balanced face these heights should be approximately equal. Clearly, the ratio between them will be affected by mid facial height, but a relative increase in lower facial height may be associated with a skeletal open bite.

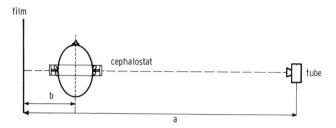

Figure 2.5 When a cephalometric radiograph is obtained, the head is held in a fixed relationship to the film and X-ray source (tube). The ratio a/b determines the enlargement of the image

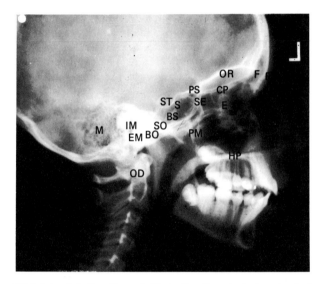

Figure 2.6 A lateral skull radiograph illustrating the principal anatomical features:

BO	= basi-occiput	N	= nasal bones
BS	= basi-sphenoid	O	= orbital margins
CP	= cribriform plate of ethmoid	OD	= odontoid process of axis
E	= ethmoid air cells	OR	= orbital roof
EM	= external acoustic meatus	PM	= pterygomaxillary fissure
F	= frontal sinus	PS	= planum sphenoidale
FN	= frontonasal suture	S	= sphenoid air sinus
HP	= hard palate	SE	= spheno-ethmoidal synchrosis
IM	= internal acoustic meatus	SO	= spheno-occipital synchrosis
M	= mastoid air cells	ST	= sella turcica, the pituitary fossa
Mx	= maxillary sinus	Z	= zygomatic process of maxilla

Transverse
The relative widths of the jaws have a bearing on the transverse relationship of the dental arches (see Chapter 8). However, there is no way, clinically or radiologically, in which these widths can be measured. Discrepancies in skeletal base width usually have to be inferred from transverse malrelationships of the arches.

Cephalometric analysis

Analysis of lateral skull radiographs allows a more detailed evaluation of facial structures than is possible from a visual assessment of facial appearance. The cephalometric lateral skull radiograph is taken with the head held in a specially designed holder (Figure 2.5) so that there is a fixed constant relationship between the patient's head, the film and the anode of the X-ray tube: the midsagittal plane of the head should be parallel to and at a fixed distance from the film so that linear measurements are magnified by a known standard amount (usually about 10%). Some experience is required if a lateral skull radiograph is to be

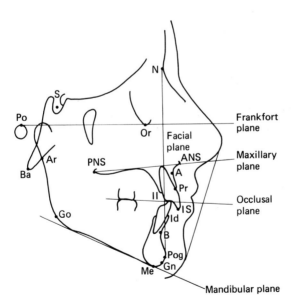

Figure 2.7 Tracing of the radiograph shown in Figure 2.6, indicating the main cephalometric landmarks (see text for definitions)

interpreted reliably. The features shown in Figure 2.6 give a key to the general anatomy. Cephalometric landmarks can then be located (Figure 2.7). The appearance of each landmark can vary appreciably between patients and some are much more difficult to identify reliably than are others. If the film is over-exposed it can be very difficult to locate the fine bony detail on the skeletal profile.

Definitions of landmarks (Figure 2.7)
Note: definitions using 'lowest' or 'highest' assume that the radiograph is orientated so that the Frankfort plane is horizontal.

Anterior nasal spine (ANS). The point of the bony nasal spine. The vertical level can be fixed quite reliably but the anteroposterior location may be difficult: the tip of the spine is thin and it may be overlaid by nasal cartilages which are nearly of the same radio-opacity. Harvold recommended the use of points on the lower and upper contours of the spine where it was 3 mm thick. These may be more reliable than the traditional ANS, but they may still be difficult to locate because the upper and lower margins of the spine are not always distinct.

Articulare (Ar). The point of intersection of the projection of the surface of the neck of the condyle and the inferior surface of the basi-occiput.

Basion (Ba). The most posterior inferior point in the midline on the basi-occiput. This marks the posterior limit of the midline cranial base and lies on the anterior rim of foramen magnum.

Gnathion (Gn). The most anterior, inferior point on the bony symphysis of the mandible. It is located where the bisector of the angle between the facial line (NPog) and the mandibular plane (through menton and tangent to the angle of the mandible) intersects the outline of the symphysis

Gonion (Go). The most posterior, inferior point on the angle of the mandible. It is located by drawing tangents to the angle of the mandible through menton and through articulare. Gonion lies where the bisector of the angle formed by these two tangents intersects the mandibular outline. This point may be used in drawing the mandibular plane and gonial angle. Where the outlines of the two sides do not coincide an 'average' outline should be drawn and the constructions related to this.

Incision inferius (II). The tip of the crown of the most prominent mandibular incisor.

Incision superius (IS). The tip of the crown of the most prominent maxillary incisor.

Infradentale (Id). The highest point on the alveolar crest labial to the most prominent lower incisor.

Menton (Me). The lowermost point on the mandibular symphysis.

Nasion (N). The most anterior point on the frontonasal suture.

Orbitale (Or). The most inferior point on the margin of the orbit. Strictly speaking, the left orbit should be used and some orthodontists use a radio-opaque pointer, or fix a marker to the skin before the radiograph is taken, to indicate this. When this is not done and two orbital borders are shown, the midpoint should be taken. Orbitale is difficult to locate with accuracy.

Pogonion (Pog). The most anterior point of the bony chin.

Point A (A). Also known as subspinale, this is the deepest point on the maxillary profile between the anterior nasal spine and the alveolar crest. It can be difficult to locate if the maxillary profile is not clear: there may be a thin spine of bone extending downwards in the midline from the anterior nasal spine, or the shadow of the cheek can be superimposed. Point A is used to indicate the anterior limit of the maxillary base but it is not very reliable in this respect because the bone in this region remodels to some extent with orthodontic tooth movement, quite apart from the problems of locating the point. However, in spite of these difficulties, point A continues to be used because no entirely satisfactory alternative has been proposed.

Point B (B). Also known as supramentale, this is the mandibular point that corresponds to point A on the maxilla; however, it is more reliable. It is the deepest point on the concavity of the mandibular profile between the point of the chin and the alveolar crest. If the curvature is gentle, the vertical level of point B may be difficult to fix, but this is not usually very important because it is used to measure anteroposterior jaw relationships.

Porion (Po). The highest point on the bony external acoustic meatus. If both sides are visible, the midpoint is taken. As already mentioned, Po can be very difficult to locate reliably. A useful guide is that the upper borders of the external acoustic meatus should be on the same level as the articulating surfaces of the mandibular condyles, although these, too, are difficult to locate. Others have suggested using the highest point on the earpost of the cephalostat, although this may vary with soft-tissue compression of the ear.

Posterior nasal spine (PNS). The tip of the PNS can usually be seen unless unerupted molars obscure it. The outline of the palate gives a good indication of its vertical level and allows the maxillary plane to be drawn in. A line through the most inferior point on the pterygomaxillary fissure, perpendicular to the maxillary plane, indicates the anteroposterior location of the PNS.

Prosthion (Pr). The lowest point on the alveolar crest labial to the most prominent upper central incisor.

Sella (S). The midpoint of the sella turcica.

Reference lines and planes (Figure 2.7)
Cephalometric measurements will be described with the analyses, but certain widely used reference planes (or more correctly 'lines' as we are dealing with a two-dimensional representation) will be described here. A very large number of reference lines in the skull are described in the anthropological literature, but only a few of direct orthodontic importance will be mentioned.

Facial line (or plane). Nasion–pogonion. It indicates the general orientation of the facial profile.

Frankfort plane. Porion–orbitale. This plane is described as being horizontal when the head is in a free postural position. In fact, there is considerable individual variation. This, together with the unreliability of its end-points and the fact that it represents no single coherent anatomical structure, means that there are serious reservations about its use as a reference structure.

Mandibular plane (Mn). A variety of lines has been used to indicate the orientation of the body of the mandible, but it probably makes little difference which is selected. The simplest to locate is the line from menton, tangent to the lower border of the mandible at the angle. The line Go–Gn is used by many but requires the construction of both points.

Maxillary plane (Mx). This line through the anterior and posterior nasal spines indicates the orientation of the palate. Where the anterior nasal spine curves upwards above the level of the nasal floor, it may be better to draw the maxillary plane through PNS parallel to the nasal floor.

Occlusal plane. Various definitions are offered. It may be represented by the line that passes through the occlusion of the mesial cusps of the most anterior permanent molars and halfway between

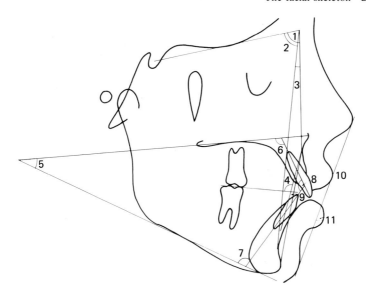

Figure 2.8 A cephalometric analysis

	Norms		This case
	Mean	Range (±)	
1. SNA	82°	3	79
2. SNB	79°	3	72
3. ANB	3°	1	7
4. AB/FOP	90°	5	100
5. A/B perp. FOP (Wit's)	0 mm	3	8
6. Max./Mand. planes (MM)	27°	5	29
7. UI/Max. Plane	108°	5	110
8. LI/Mand.Plane	92°	5	102
9. UI/LI	133°	10	119
10. LI to A–Pog	0 mm	2	+4
11. Upper lip to aesthetic plane	0 mm	–	+1
12. Lower lip to aesthetic plane	0 mm	–	+4

Comments: Angle SNA is low but just within normal range, while SNB is
definitely low. Angle ANB at 7 degrees indicates a definite Class II skeletal
pattern and this is corroborated by the large angle between the line A–B and
the functional occlusal plane (FOP). Another method of examining the skeletal
pattern is Wit's analysis: measuring the difference at the FOP of perpendiculars
from A and B points. In this case a significant Class II discrepancy is shown. A
normal reading would be 0 mm for females and B perp. +1 mm for males. The
upper incisors are at an average inclination to the maxillary plane, while the
lower incisors are proclined with the incisor edges in advance of the A–Pog line,
indicating some dento-alveolar compensation for the Class II skeletal pattern.
Vertically, the jaw relationships are within normal limits. The lips were parted
when the radiograph was taken, with the lower lip rather full and everted lying
in advance of the aesthetic plane. It is important to assess clinically whether this
correctly portrays the habitual lip posture

the tips of the upper and lower central incisors. It is preferable to use a line following the occlusion of the molar and premolar teeth. This is known as the functional occlusal plane (FOP).

Many landmarks are a compromise between anatomical validity and the possibility of identification. For example, points A and B which are meant to represent maxillary and mandibular skeletal base, respectively, are affected to a limited extent by tooth movement and alveolar remodelling. Thus cephalometric measurements must be interpreted with caution and too much emphasis should not be placed on minor variations in their values. If a cephalometric measurement is to have any meaning it is necessary to know the normal range of that measurement within the population group from which the patient comes (Figure 2.8). Even if one measurement is beyond the normal range, it may be compensated for by other features and so it is necessary to look for a general pattern. The basic question is whether there is evidence of skeletal malrelationships and whether or not there has been dento-alveolar compensation. It is then possible to decide about the tooth movements that would be necessary to correct the arch malrelationships; and whether tipping movements (obtainable with a removable appliance) or controlled apical movement (requiring fixed appliances) will be appropriate. Where the skeletal discrepancy is severe, surgical correction may be considered.

Treatment planning must never be undertaken using cephalometric analysis in isolation: the stability and aesthetic acceptability of the intended tooth movements can be fully evaluated only by reference to the soft-tissue pattern and facial appearance of the living patient.

Measurement from lateral skull radiographs

The relevant anatomical lines should be traced on to good quality tracing paper using a sharp, hard pencil. A very large number of cephalometric measurements has been proposed but, for the clinician, those shown in Figure 2.8 give a comprehensive view of skeletal and dentoskeletal relationships.

Electronic digitizers linked to a computer with a suitable software package loaded are used increasingly for cephalometric analysis. Such a system speeds the whole process while facilitating the application of more than one method of analysis. This is particularly useful in cases requiring orthognathic surgery. The software will allow manipulation of the image on the monitor to assess the effects of different surgical procedures. Newly developed systems allow the merger of video-captured images of the patient together with the appropriate radiograph, but are still expensive and await proof of their usefulness and validity before being universally adopted.

The interpretation of cephalometric measurements

Points A and B are taken to represent the anterior limits of the tooth-bearing areas of the maxilla and mandible. This relationship is usually assessed by reference to the anterior cranial base (S–N line). Angles SNA and SNB measure the prognathism, or projection in relation to the cranial base, of the maxilla and mandible. The difference between these (angle ANB) gives an indication of the jaw relationships as follows:

Angle ANB	Skeletal class
2–4°	I
greater than 4°	II
less than 2°	III

This value can be misleading if the position of N is unusual, but a warning of this may be given by a value of SNA that is unusually large or small. An alternative method of assessing the jaw relationship is to measure the angle between A and B and the functional occlusal plane (FOP). Perpendicular lines may also be dropped from these points to the occlusal plane (Wit's analysis). A problem with both measurements is that the orientation of the FOP varies greatly between individuals and can change with growth and treatment. However, they offer a useful check on the information given by angle ANB: if different evaluations of the skeletal pattern are contradictory, then each should be interpreted with caution and a final judgement on skeletal relationships made from clinical observations.

As with direct clinical observation, the anterior height of the intermaxillary space may be estimated from the angle of the mandibular plane to the Frankfort plane, but as the latter is often difficult to locate on a radiograph the maxillary plane (ANS–PNS) is often used instead. On average, the Frankfort and maxillary planes are parallel to one another but they may diverge appreciably in some individuals.

Dentoskeletal relationships

The inclinations of the upper incisors to the maxillary plane and of the lower incisors to the mandibular plane give an indication of whether or not any dento-alveolar compensation for antero-posterior skeletal discrepancies has taken place. They also give a guide to the type of tooth movements that will be required to correct incisor malrelationships. The distance of the most prominent lower incisor from the line between point A and the chin point (pogonion) is a guide to the position of the lower incisors relative to the lower skeletal profile. It is simpler to obtain a good incisor relationship and the appearance is usually better if the lower incisor edge lies close to the A–Pog line, than if it is far from it. However, this line should not be regarded as a treatment goal to the positioning of the lower incisors because it offers no guide to the position of stability.

The angle between the upper and lower incisors is related to the depth of overbite (except in Class III cases). A wide inter-incisor angle is usually associated with a deep overbite and if at the end of treatment this angle is too large, the overbite will usually deepen and may become traumatic.

The soft-tissue profile

Various cephalometric assessments of the soft-tissue profile have been proposed. It must be recognized that none of these can give guidance as to whether a particular face is attractive or not and such measurements are of very little diagnostic value. However, they may help in describing a patient's facial appearance. Perhaps the most useful of these is the Aesthetic Line which touches the tip of the nose and the tip of the chin. It has been maintained that the facial appearance is more likely to be pleasing when the lips lie close to this line. Another indicator is the nasolabial angle: ideally the nasolabial angle should be in the order of 110°. Too wide a nasolabial angle often gives a rather poor facial appearance. Careful consideration should be given to the management of patients with a tendency towards a more obtuse nasiolabial angle: reduction of an overjet, particularly with a fixed appliance, can have undesirable effects on the lip profile.

Racial variation

Note the norm figures given above have been derived from Caucasian groups and should not be applied to other racial groups.

Chapter 3

Soft-tissue morphology and behaviour

The soft tissues

Traditionally the soft tissues considered to be of greatest relevance to orthodontics have been the lips and the tongue, with the emphasis being placed on their respective functions during swallowing. However, it is important to remember that other soft tissues of the mouth may also have a role in the aetiology of malocclusion and the outcome of orthodontic treatment.

The lips

The lips may be described as being either competent or incompetent.

Competent lips

In this situation the lips are held together easily, with minimal activity of the circumoral musculature, forming an anterior oral seal when the mandible is in the rest position (Figure 3.1a).

In patients where the lips have the potential to meet easily together, but are held apart, the term potentially competent may be applied. This may be found in patients where prominent upper incisors rest between the lips or where nasal obstruction encourages mouth breathing.

Incompetent lips

In this situation, with minimal activity of the circumoral musculature and the mandible in the rest position, the lips are held apart. In the absence of any neuromuscular deficit, such as that found in cerebral palsy, this is usually due to an imbalance between the anterior lower face height and the length of the upper and lower

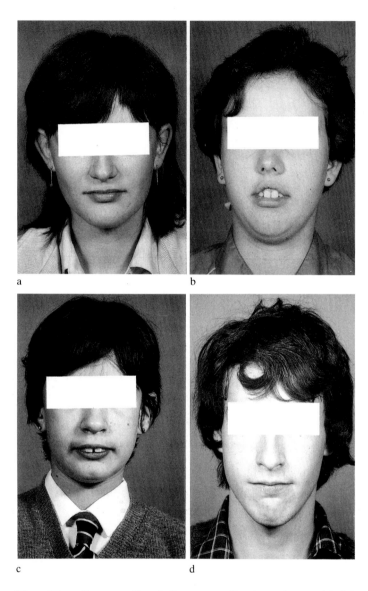

Figure 3.1 a, Competent lips. b, Incompetent lips due to increased facial height. c, Incompetent lips due to severe anteroposterior skeletal discrepancy. d, Incompetent lips held together by muscular effort – note the puckering of the skin over the chin, signifying mentalis muscle activity

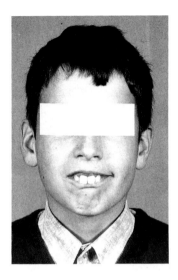

Figure 3.2 Tongue-to-lower-lip oral seal. Note that the upper lip plays no part in forming an anterior oral seal. The activity of the lower lip will hinder the overjet reduction

lips (Figure 3.1b) or a severe anteroposterior discrepancy (Figure 3.1c).

The degree of incompetence varies between individuals, depending on both their skeletal and dental architecture. Mild or moderately incompetent lips may be held together with muscular effort. This can be recognized by the puckering of the skin over the chin due to the contraction of the mentalis muscle (Figure 3.1d). In more severe cases the patient will have great difficulty in achieving even transitory lip contact.

Lip exercises (which are prescribed by some clinicians for use with certain types of functional appliances) will not increase lip length, but they may encourage the development of a neuromuscular habit that brings the lips together. Such changes may be difficult to distinguish from those that are often seen to occur naturally as the child matures.

Significance of lips

It has been suggested that the lower lip has an important role in the development of a malocclusion, in treatment to correct a malocclusion and in the long-term stability of the corrected malocclusion. The form of the lower lip may guide the path of the erupting permanent incisors. In patients with a reduced anterior lower face height, the lower lip may direct the erupting maxillary

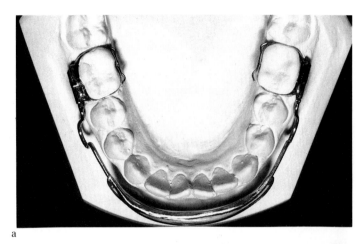

a

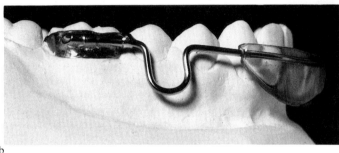

b

Figure 3.3 A lip bumper being used to harness muscular forces from the lower lip in order to move lower molars distally: a, occlusal view; b, right buccal view

incisors down its inner surface and contribute to the establishment of a Class II Division 2 malocclusion, or alternatively it may guide the incisors labially to produce a Class II Division 1 malocclusion. Of course, the developmental position of the incisors is also an important contributory factor and the interrelationship between soft and hard tissues is complex. Clinically it is found that where the lips are full and everted both the upper and lower labial segments are more often proclined (bimaxillary proclination), whereas in individuals with more vertically positioned or straight lips the upper and lower labial segments are more often retroclined (bimaxillary retroclination).

During treatment of a Class II Division 1 malocclusion, the presence of a vigorous muscular activity of the lower lip maintaining an anterior oral seal to the tongue may make overjet reduction difficult (Figures 3.2 and 10.2a). On occasions such muscular activity of the lower lip may be harnessed by means of a lip bumper to help move lower teeth distally (Figure 3.3a,b).

The long-term stability of a corrected Class II Division 1 malocclusion relies on the lower lip covering the incisal third of the labial surface of the upper incisors to control their position (see Figure 10.2b). If this treatment aim cannot be achieved there is a risk that without permanent or semi-permanent retention of upper incisor position the overjet will re-establish.

The tongue

The tongue adapts to the form of the oral cavity. In the infant the tongue lies between the gum pads in contact with the lips and cheeks. Feeding and swallowing take place with the tongue in this forward position. As the teeth erupt oral function changes, mastication is established and there is a gradual maturation of tongue activity from an infant to a more adult pattern. This is usually complete by the time the deciduous dentition has become established. However, for a small number of individuals the infantile pattern of behaviour may persist and influence the position of incisor teeth.

In the past, much attention has been paid to the activities of the tongue and lips during swallowing and their supposedly irrevocable effect on tooth position. However, recent evidence would suggest that tooth position is influenced more by light continuous forces (such as are found with the soft tissues at rest) than by heavy intermittent forces (such as are found during swallowing), and while we cannot ignore the effect that an atypical swallow may have on tooth position, it is probably less important than was believed hitherto.

Muscle balance

The teeth occupy a position of balance determined by the interaction between the tongue and lips, the jaw relationship and occlusal forces. If the position of the teeth is to be altered and remain stable, another position of balance must be sought. Alteration of the balance of soft-tissue forces, by relieving the

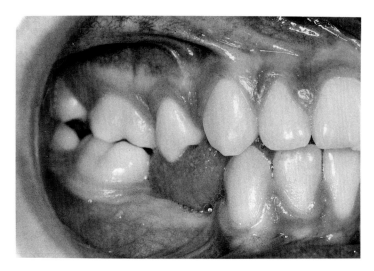

Figure 3.4 Lateral spread of the tongue following loss of the first and second deciduous molars preventing substantial mesial movement of the lower first permanent molar. Note also that there has been no over-eruption of the opposing premolar

pressures of the cheeks and lips while allowing the tongue to expand the dental arches laterally and anteroposteriorly, is deliberately attempted by the exponents of some myofunctional appliances (see Chapter 16).

Lateral spread of the tongue, especially in the lower arch, has been suggested as the mechanism that prevents as much mesial movement of the first permanent molar when both deciduous molars have been extracted as when a single deciduous second molar has been lost (Figure 3.4).

Adaptive tongue behaviour

The tongue will usually work in conjunction with the lower lip to form an anterior oral seal. This may be found in different circumstances, as outlined below.

Incompetent lips
Where the lips are incompetent and habitually parted, an anterior oral seal may be obtained by contact between the tongue and lower lip. This will be associated with an incomplete overbite and

some upper incisor proclination. If orthodontic treatment allows a normal lip-to-lip anterior oral seal to be established, the result should be stable.

Increases in overjet
A large overjet such as is found in a Class II skeletal pattern will lead to an anterior oral seal by tongue/lower lip contact. The features are similar to those associated with incompetent lips (above).

Incomplete overbite (or anterior open bite)
If the overbite is incomplete, due for example to a digit-sucking habit or an increased lower face height, the tongue will come forwards over the lower incisors. As with all adaptive characteristics this will spontaneously revert to normal on correction of the malocclusion.

Primary atypical tongue behaviour
Rarely there is an inborn atypical pattern of neuromuscular activity by which the tongue remains in its more infantile position, and pushes actively forwards during swallowing (an endogenous tongue thrust). This can produce both an increase in overjet and a reduction in overbite. Clinically it is difficult to distinguish between the atypical (endogenous) and the adaptive tongue behaviour. However, the difference is important since correction of the former is likely to be unstable. The following guidelines may help in recognizing atypical tongue behaviour:

• The tongue is thrust forwards more forcibly than with adaptive patterns and the amount of circumoral contraction seems to be greater than would have been expected from the degree of lip incompetence.
• The incompleteness of the overbite is greater than is found with adaptive tongue behaviour associated with lip incompetence or a large overjet. Remember that digit-sucking habits or increased anterior skeletal face height may be associated with a similar vertical incisor arrangement.

Other oral tissues

Fraenum

The upper labial fraenum has been implicated in the persistence of a midline diastema (see Chapter 6).

The lower midline labial fraenum may retain its point of attachment high on the gingival margin of the lower incisors, and the pull exerted by this may lead to the formation of a Stillman's cleft. While this, in itself, will not contribute to a malocclusion, from a periodontal point of view the poor prognosis may influence the orthodontic extraction pattern, especially in the adult.

Periodontal tissues

The mucosa surrounding the teeth remodels at a much slower rate than the alveolar bone. The supracrestal periodontal fibres have been shown to stretch when a tooth is derotated, and take up to 9 months to reorganize fully. This has implications for the length of retention following treatment (see Chapter 13).

Reduction of an overjet using a removal appliance may be hindered by an accumulation of the soft tissues palatal to the upper incisors. Unless provision is made for the soft tissues to build up by judicious trimming of the baseplate, tooth movement can be brought to a halt, and the soft tissues ulcerate and cause pain as they become trapped between the baseplate and the teeth (see Chapter 14).

Chapter 4

Normal occlusion – development and function

Development of normal occlusion

Occlusal development may be divided into five stages:

Stage 1. Birth to establishment of deciduous dentition.
Stage 2. Deciduous dentition to early mixed dentition.
Stage 3. Early mixed dentition to late mixed dentition.
Stage 4. Late mixed dentition to permanent dentition.
Stage 5. Permanent dentition.

While these stages form a convenient basis for description, occlusal development should be considered a continuous process.

Stage 1. Birth to establishment of deciduous dentition

At birth, the maxillary and mandibular gum pads have 20 segmented elevations corresponding to the unerupted deciduous teeth. The elevation for the second deciduous molars are poorly defined at birth and are not properly present until the age of 5 months. The groove that marks the distal margin of the canine segment continues into the buccal sulcus and is called the 'lateral sulcus'.

The upper arch is horseshoe-shaped and the vault of the palate is very shallow. The alveolar part is separated on its palatal side from the hard palate by a continuous horizontal groove known as the 'dental or gingival groove'. The lower arch is U-shaped and the gum pad anteriorly is slightly everted labially.

With the mandible in its physiological rest position the gum pads are apart, with the tongue filling the space between them and projecting against the lips anteriorly, the lower lip forming the principal boundary to the front of the oral cavity. The upper lip appears to be very short at this age.

The gum pads rarely come into occlusion. The maxillary gum pad overlaps the mandibular both buccally and labially, corresponding to the ultimate occlusal relationship of the teeth (Figure

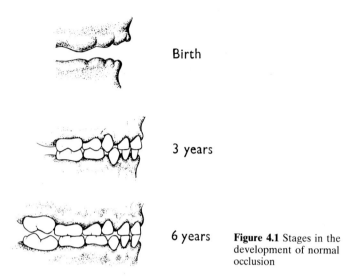

Birth

3 years

6 years **Figure 4.1** Stages in the development of normal occlusion

4.1). The gum pads at birth are not sufficiently wide to accommodate the developing incisors which are crowded and rotated in their crypts. During the first year of life the gum pads grow rapidly, especially laterally. This ultimately permits incisors to erupt in good alignment, helped by pressure from the tongue and lips.

Neonatal teeth
Occasionally a child is born with teeth already erupted. These are termed neonatal teeth. They are usually normal teeth from the deciduous series, but have little root development. This, in turn, means that they are often quite mobile, but there is no indication to remove them unless they are interfering with feeding (usually causing discomfort to the mother during breast feeding) or if they are so loose that there is a danger of exfoliation.

The deciduous dentition (Table 4.1)

Eruption of the lower central incisors begins at about 6 months of age. It should be recognized that the timing of eruption is very variable and a range of 6 months on either side of the representative figures given in Table 4.1 is commonplace. Usually by the age of 2½ years all the deciduous teeth have erupted (Figure 4.1).

Table 4.1 Typical ages of eruption and mesiodistal widths of the deciduous teeth

	Time of eruption (months)	Mesiodistal width (mm)
Maxillary teeth		
Central incisor	8	6.5
Lateral incisor	9	5.0
Canine	18	6.5
First molar	14	7.0
Second molar	24	8.5
Mandibular teeth		
Central incisor	6	4.0
Lateral incisor	7	4.5
Canine	16	5.5
First molar	12	8.0
Second molar	20	9.5

Notes:
1. Mesiodistal widths vary by up to 20% on either side of the figures given.
2. Calcification of the deciduous teeth begins between 4 and 6 months *in utero*.
3. Root formation is complete between 12 and 18 months after eruption.
4. There is often a difference of a few weeks between tooth eruption on the left and right sides.
5. Usually the lower teeth erupt ahead of their upper counterparts.

Points to notice at 2½ years
1. The incisors are more vertical than their permanent successors and they are often spaced.
2. There may be spacing distal to the lower canines and mesial to the upper canines (the so-called 'primate spacing').
3. The distal surfaces of the second deciduous molars should end in line with each other (termed the 'flush terminal plane').

Stage 2. Deciduous dentition to early mixed dentition
(Table 4.2)

At the age of 6 years permanent teeth, usually the first molars or lower central incisors, start to erupt. As in the case of the deciduous teeth, eruption times and the order of eruption are very variable and a range of 18 months on either side of the figures given in Table 4.2 is not unusual.

The permanent incisors

The permanent incisors develop lingual to the roots of the deciduous incisors (Figure 4.2a). Space for these teeth, which are larger than their deciduous predecessors, is provided by:

Table 4.2 Typical ages of eruption and mesiodistal widths of the permanent teeth

	Time of eruption (years)	Mesiodistal width (mm)
Maxillary teeth		
Central incisor	7.5	8.5
Lateral incisor	8.5	6.5
Canine	11.5	8.0
First premolar	10.0	7.0
Second premolar	11.0	6.5
First molar	6.0	10.0
Second molar	12.0	9.5
Mandibular teeth		
Central incisor	6.5	5.5
Lateral incisor	7.5	6.0
Canine	10.0	7.0
First premolar	10.5	7.0
Second premolar	11.0	7.0
First molar	6.0	11.0
Second molar	12.0	10.5

Notes:
1. The figures given both for eruption times and for mesiodistal widths commonly vary by up to 20% on either side of the figures given.
2 Calcification dates are variable but the permanent teeth have usually started to calcify as follows:
  At Birth 6̲
         6
  By 6 months 1̲ 3̲
           123
  By 2 years 2̲4̲
         4
  By 4 years 5̲ 7̲
        5 7
  Between 8 and 14 years 8̲
               8
3. Root formation is normally completed 2–3 years after eruption.

- Utilization of existing spacing between the deciduous incisors.
- A growth increase in intercanine width which takes place during the eruption of the incisors.
- The upper permanent incisors are more proclined and thus form a larger arch than the deciduous incisors.

Notes:
(a) If the deciduous incisor root is not resorbed normally, the permanent incisor may be deflected lingually (Figure 4.2b).
(b) The upper lateral incisors in their developmental position are overlapped by the central incisors (Figure 4.2a). They escape as the central incisors erupt. However, if there is insufficient growth in arch width they may be trapped in this palatal position.

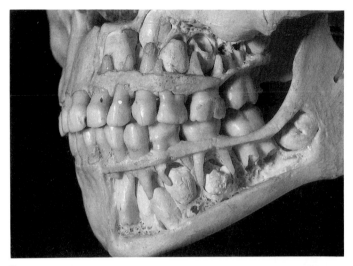

a

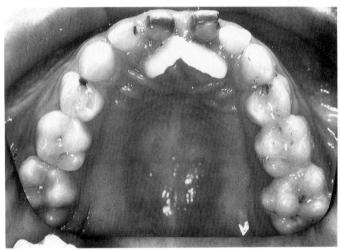

b

Figure 4.2 a, Developmental positions of the permanent incisors. Note that the permanent incisors develop lingual to the roots of the deciduous incisors and that the upper lateral incisors are overlapped by the central incisors and canines. b, Palatal eruption of permanent upper central incisors. Note retained deciduous predecessors

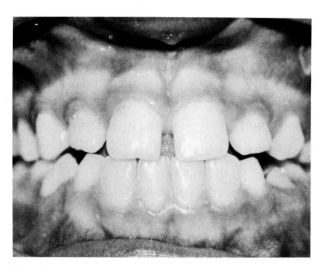

Figure 4.3 The 'ugly duckling' stage

(c) When the upper incisors erupt they are frequently distally inclined so that there is a median diastema (Figure 4.3). This is the 'ugly duckling' stage and is due to the incisor roots being crowded mesially by the permanent canine crowns. When the permanent canines erupt the median diastema (physiological spacing) will usually close. This natural developmental stage should not be mistaken for a malocclusion and treatment must not be undertaken to close the diastema before the permanent canines erupt.

There is usually a small growth spurt associated with the eruption of the first permanent molars leading to an increase in face height, and a growth in width across the canine region to accommodate the larger permanent incisor teeth. This growth in width usually ceases at around the age of 9 years.

The permanent molars

These are guided into position by the distal surfaces of the second deciduous molars. In a normal occlusal relationship the flush terminal plane of the deciduous molars brings the first permanent molars into cusp-to-cusp contact.

Stage 3. Early mixed dentition to late mixed dentition

After the rapid and dramatic changes that occur during the transition from deciduous to permanent incisors, and the eruption of the first permanent molars, there is a lull in occlusal development for about 12–18 months. The start of the next stage is usually signalled by the eruption of the mandibular canines and maxillary first premolars.

Stage 4. Late mixed dentition to permanent dentition

During this phase the remaining deciduous teeth are shed and replaced by their permanent successors. The discrepancy between the mesiodistal widths of the deciduous molars and the premolars creates space in both arches and is termed the 'leeway space'. The leeway space is greater in the lower arch than the upper arch, and this allows the lower permanent molar to move forward further than the upper molar and establish a Class I molar relationship, i.e. the mesiobuccal cusp of the maxillary first permanent molar occludes with the midbuccal groove of the lower first permanent molar. The second permanent molars should be guided directly into occlusion by the distal surfaces of the first permanent molars.

The upper permanent molars develop in the maxillary tuberosity with their occlusal surfaces facing distally and buccally as well as occlusally. Posterior growth in maxillary length is necessary to allow them to rotate forwards and downwards into the line of the arch. The mandibular molars develop under the anterior border of the ascending ramus of the mandible. Growth in mandibular length, which involves resorption on the anterior margin of the ascending ramus, is necessary if the tooth is to have room to erupt.

Stage 5. Permanent dentition

The variability of presence and morphology of third molars means that these teeth are rarely considered in descriptions of occlusion. Angle's classification was based on the relationship of the first molars, a normal or Class I molar relationship described as above. More recently Andrews has described six keys to a normal occlusion, i.e. these are features that are commonly found in non-orthodontic, well ordered, occlusions. They form a basis for identifying deviations from a normal occlusion' and a treatment goal for orthodontic correction.

Key I.   Molar relationship:

(a) The distal surface of the distal marginal ridge of the upper first permanent molar contacts and occludes with the mesial surface of the mesial marginal ridge of the lower second molar.

(b) The mesiobuccal cusp of the upper first permanent molar falls within the groove between the mesial and middle cusps of the lower first permanent molar.

(c) The mesiolingual cusp of the upper first permanent molar seats in the central fossa of the lower first permanent molar.

Key II.   Crown angulation:

The gingival portion of the long axis of each crown is distal to the occlusal portion of that axis, i.e. each tooth crown has a mesiodistal tip and this varies with each tooth.

Key III.   Crown inclination:

For upper incisors the gingival portion of the labial surface of the crown is lingual to the incisal portion.

For all other teeth the gingival portion of the labial or buccal surface of the crown is labial or buccal to the incisal/occlusal portion.

This is called labiolingual torque.

Key IV.   Rotations:

There should be no rotations.

Key V.   Contacts:

Provided there are no genuine tooth-size discrepancies, there should be tight contact points.

Key VI.   Curve of Spee:

This is measured from incisors to molars and should not exceed a depth of 1.5 mm.

This is a fairly full description of a static occlusal relationship, to which Roth has added some functional goals for occlusion:

- Centric occlusion and centric relation should coincide.
- Occlusal forces should be directed down the long axes of the posterior teeth.
- There should be 0.005 in (0.1270 mm) space between the anterior teeth when in occlusion.
- In lateral and protrusive mandibular movements the canines and incisors disclude the posterior teeth.

He calls this a mutually protective occlusal scheme whereby the posterior teeth protect the anterior teeth in occlusion, and the anterior teeth protect the posterior teeth during mandibular excursions.

While Roth, and other orthodontists, favour mutually protective (also referred to as canine-guided) occlusion as a functional goal, it must be emphasized that there is little scientific evidence to support either canine guidance, or the alternative occlusal philosophy of group function, as the ideal functional occlusion. Furthermore, concerns that a poor functional occlusion may predispose a patient to temporomandibular joint dysfunction (TMJD) have yet to be proved. It is likely that this may be one of a constellation of factors operating simultaneously which create the problem.

Nevertheless prevention of the possible development of TMJD is almost always given as a reason for correction of a mandibular displacement associated with a crossbite. Although the position of maximal occlusion should be a position of centric relation, in a number of patients, due to occlusal interferences (premature contacts), the mandible is displaced during its path of closure from the rest to the occlusal position. Displacements may be lateral (e.g. if there is a unilateral crossbite), anterior (e.g. if there are instanding incisors), or (rarely) posterior (e.g. if there has been loss of posterior teeth and there is a Class II Division 2 incisor relationship). In addition, with the maturing of the occlusion in the adult there is an underlying tendency for the position of maximal occlusion and centric relation to diverge (see Chapter 12).

When examining the patient it is important to distinguish between deviations and displacements of the mandible during closure from the rest position into the position of maximal occlusion. Deviations are basically habit postures often disguising an underlying overjet, whereas a displacement is directly related to an occlusal interference and usually occurs late in the process of closing into the position of maximal occlusion.

Changes in the permanent occlusion

The eruption into occlusion of all the permanent teeth (except the third molars) between the ages of 12 and 14 years does not mark the end of occlusal change.

An increase in incisor crowding
This may be associated with mandibular growth rotations and corresponding dento-alveolar adaptation as described earlier.

It has also been suggested that mesial drift of buccal teeth may contribute to this late crowding. Mesial drift is observed when the continuity of the arch is broken by extraction of teeth but the cause is not understood. The following explanations have been offered:

- It is a natural growth tendency in the human.
- Crowded teeth, particularly third molars, exert a forward pressure on the other teeth. It should be noted, however, that mesial drift occurs even where third molars are developmentally absent.
- The anterior component of force: this arises because the upper and lower teeth are slightly mesially inclined. Vertical occlusal loading produces an intrusive force and a small anterior component of force which could be responsible for mesial drift. However, the evidence in support of this theory is insubstantial.

It is disappointing to realize that similar changes in the dental arrangement can occur even following orthodontic treatment. There appear to be no good prognostic indicators of an occlusion which will stay stable in the late teenage years and onwards or one which will deteriorate.

Chapter 5

Malocclusion

A malocclusion is defined as an irregularity of the teeth or a malrelationship of the dental arches beyond the accepted range of normal. Thus malocclusions are for the most part variations around the normal and are a representation of biological variability. Biological variation is expressed elsewhere in the body, but minor irregularities are more readily noticed and recorded in the dentition and so have attracted greater attention with an associated demand for treatment. The majority of malocclusions are primarily of hereditary causation although environmental factors, e.g. the unplanned extraction of teeth, may also contribute.

There is evidence that the prevalence of malocclusion is increasing, particularly in developed communities. This increase may in part reflect an underlying evolutionary trend towards shorter jaws and fewer teeth, but it is probably largely the result of an increase in the genetic variability of these populations brought about by intermixture of racial groups. It has been proposed by Begg that one reason for the increase in the prevalence of crowding is that there is now little approximal or occlusal attrition of the teeth. In primitive people living on a coarse diet an appreciable reduction in the mesiodistal widths of erupted teeth occurs due to attrition. This loss of tooth substance, which can amount to several millimetres in each quadrant, would reduce a tendency to crowding. Unfortunately, there is little solid evidence to support this view.

Malocclusions may be associated with one or more of the following:

● Malposition of individual teeth.
● Malrelationship of the dental arches.

Malocclusion of individual teeth

A tooth may occupy a position other than normal by being:

1. *Tipped.* The tooth apex is normally placed but the crown incorrectly positioned. Teeth may be tipped laterally (termed 'angulation') or may be tipped labiopalatally (termed 'inclination').
2. *Displaced.* Both apex and crown are incorrectly positioned.
3. *Rotated.* The tooth is rotated around its long axis.
4. *In infra-occlusion.* The tooth has not reached the occlusal level.
5. *In supra-occlusion.* The tooth has erupted past the occlusal level.
6. *Transposed.* Two teeth have reversed their positions. An example of this might be an upper canine and first premolar.

Teeth that are tilted or displaced are described according to the direction of the malposition; for example, an incisor may be labially inclined (or proclined), lingually inclined (or retroclined), mesially angulated, or distally angulated. Similar terms may be applied to displacements. Rotations are probably best described by the approximal surface that is furthest from the line of the arch and the direction it faces; for example, a rotated upper incisor is described as mesiolabially rotated if the mesial aspect is out of the line of the arch while a similar rotation would be described as distopalatal if the distal aspect was palatally positioned.

Malrelationship of the dental arches

Malrelationships of the arches may occur in any of the three planes of space: anteroposterior, vertical or transverse. The aetiology and treatment of vertical and transverse malrelationships are dealt with in Chapter 8. The classifications of malocclusion described in this text are based on anteroposterior relationships as described below. The aetiology and treatment of these malrelationships are dealt with in Chapters 9–12.

Classification of malocclusion

For convenience of description, it is useful to have some classification that will divide up the wide range of malocclusions into a small number of groups. Many classifications have been proposed but the one that is universally recognized is Angle's classification, which is based on arch relationship in the sagittal plane. The key relationship in Angle's classification is that of the first permanent molars: in normal occlusions, the anterior buccal groove of the lower first permanent molar should occlude with the anterior buccal cusp of the upper first permanent molar (see Figure 1.1). If the first molars have drifted, allowance must be made for this before the occlusion is classified.

Angle's classification

Class I. Malocclusions in which the lower first permanent molar is within one-half cusp width of its correct relationship to the upper first permanent molar (Figure 5.1). This arch relationship is sometimes known as 'neutro-occlusion'.

Class II. The lower arch is at least one-half cusp width posterior to the correct relationship with the upper arch, judged by the first molar relationship (Figures 5.2 and 5.3). This arch relationship is sometimes known as 'disto-occlusion'.

Class II may be further subdivided according to the inclination of the upper central incisors:
Division 1. The upper central incisors are proclined or of average inclination with an increase in overjet (Figure 5.2).
Division 2. The upper central incisors are retroclined (Figure 5.3), being less than 105° to the maxillary plane. The overjet is usually average but may be a little increased. Sometimes the upper lateral incisors are proclined, mesially inclined and mesiolabially rotated.

Class III. The lower arch is at least one-half cusp width too far forward in relation to the upper arch, judged by the first permanent molar relationship (Figure 5.4). This arch relationship is sometimes known as 'mesio-occlusion'.

A number of problems may be encountered when attempting to classify a particular malocclusion according to Angle's method:

1. The first permanent molars may have been extracted or they may have drifted following early loss of deciduous molar teeth. Where the first molars have drifted forwards as a result of early loss, due allowance should be made before classification. This is not always simple and it is well worth while looking at the general features of the occlusion and in particular at the permanent canine relationship. The upper permanent canine should occlude into the embrasure between the lower canine and first premolar. This relationship should match the first permanent molar relationship: in Class II cases, the embrasure between the lower canine and first premolar will be distal to the cusp of the upper canine, whereas in Class III cases, it will

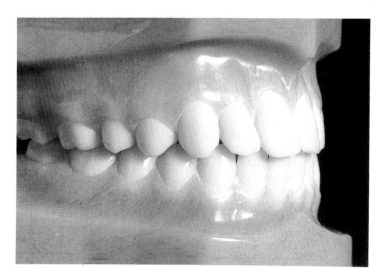

Figure 5.1 An Angle's Class I malocclusion

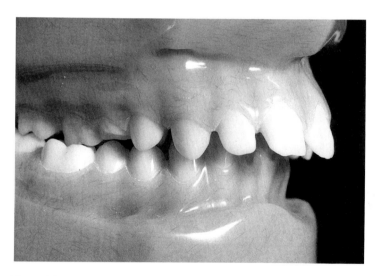

Figure 5.2 An Angle's Class II Division 1 malocclusion

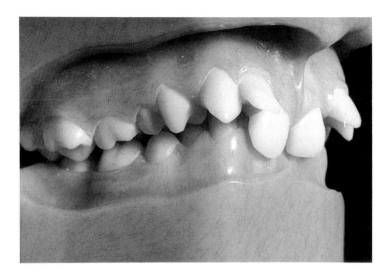

Figure 5.3 An Angle's Class II Division 2 malocclusion

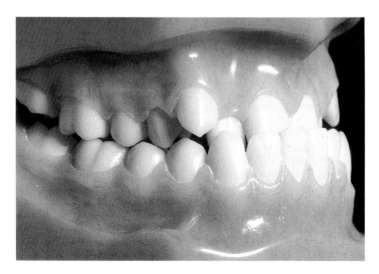

Figure 5.4 An Angle's Class III malocclusion

be too far forwards. In general, if the mólar and canine relationship match one another, the classification can be affirmed with reasonable confidence; but if they do not, care must be taken and classification may have to be undertaken on the general features of the occlusion.

2. The occlusion may differ between sides. Angle allowed for this by describing subdivisions of Class II and Class III where one side was in a normal relationship. However, it is probably more useful to classify the occlusion according to its general features.

3. It can be difficult to know where to draw the dividing line between Class I and the other classes. Here again, the final decision must rest on the general features of the occlusion. It is often helpful to look also to the position of the upper disto-buccal cusp of the first permanent molar. In a Class I relationship with good function, this normally occludes to the embrasure between the lower first and second permanent molars.

Angle considered that the first permanent molars had constant developmental relationships to their respective jaws so that, by classifying the occlusion, the skeletal pattern could also be assessed. It must be emphasized that this assumption is not correct and that the developmental positions of the teeth on the jaws may vary. Thus the occlusal and skeletal classification may not necessarily coincide.

Incisor classification

The incisor relationship does not always match the buccal segment relationship. Since much of orthodontic treatment is focused on the correction of incisor malrelationships, it is helpful to have a classification of incisor relationships (Figure 5.5). The terms used are the same but this is not Angle's classification, although it is a derivation. In clinical practice the incisor classification is usually found to be more useful than Angle's classification.

Class I. The lower incisor edges occlude with or lie immediately below the cingulum plateau (middle part of the palatal surface) of the upper central incisors (Figure 5.5a).

Class II. The lower incisor edges lie posterior to the cingulum plateau of the upper incisors.

There are two divisions to Class II malocclusion:

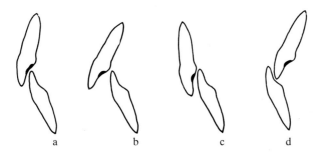

Figure 5.5 Incisor classification: a, Class I; b, Class II Division 1; c, Class II Division 2; d, Class III

Division 1. The upper central incisors are proclined or of average inclination and there is an increased overjet (Figure 5.5b).

Division 2. The upper central incisors are retroclined (less than 105° to the maxillary plane). The overjet is usually average but may be increased (Figure 5.5c).

Class III. The lower incisor edges lie anterior to the cingulum plateau of the upper incisors (Figure 5.5d). The overjet may be either reduced or reversed.

The aetiology of malocclusion

For the convenience of this discussion, the causes of malocclusion can broadly be divided into general factors and local factors .

General factors are discussed in detail in the relevant chapters and include variations in skeletal relationship (Chapter 2), disproportion between tooth and arch size that may result in either crowding or spacing (Chapter 7) and soft-tissue factors (Chapter 3).

Malocclusions may also be associated with a number of genetic and developmental disorders. Examples of this might include Down's syndrome (mongolism), hypothyroidism (cretinism), cleidocranial dysostosis and many other relatively uncommon syndromes. To maintain the brevity of the current text these will not be discussed further here. However, due to the dental importance and comparative frequency of cleft lip and palate, this condition is discussed further in Chapter 21.

Local factors are essentially habits and anomalies in the number, form and developmental positions of the teeth. In spite of their classification as local factors, their effects may be quite extensive. Local factors may coexist with one another and with any of the general factors mentioned above. They will be discussed in Chapter 6.

Local factors in the aetiology of malocclusion

It is convenient to discuss local factors under the following headings: anomalies in the number of teeth; anomalies in the form and developmental position of teeth; habits and other local factors.

Anomalies in the number of teeth

- Developmentally missing teeth.
- Early loss of deciduous teeth.
- Loss of permanent teeth.
- Retained deciduous teeth.
- Supernumerary teeth.

Developmentally missing teeth

Anodontia
The total failure of development of all teeth is a rare condition due to aplasia of the dental lamina. It is often associated with ectodermal dysplasia, an hereditary condition in which there is dry coarse skin, sparse hair, defects of the nails and absence of sweat glands. Anodontia is a prosthetic problem but it should be noted that the growth of the facial skeleton (apart from the alveolar processes of maxilla and mandible which are absent) is usually within normal limits.

Hypodontia/oligodontia
The developmental absence of a number of teeth is sometimes associated with ectodermal dysplasia, as in the case of anodontia. In these cases, the teeth that are present are often conical in form and reduced in size. These patients present a major dental problem and partial dentures or bridges are required. Osseo-integrated implants also have a major role in the oral rehabilitation of these cases. Where possible, treatment of this sort should

be delayed until the patient is old enough to maintain an excellent standard of oral hygiene while wearing a prosthesis.

Far more common than either of the conditions described above is the absence of a few teeth in an otherwise perfectly normal child. The teeth most commonly missing are third molars, upper lateral incisors, lower second premolars and upper second premolars.

Third molars. The absence of these teeth is not an orthodontic problem. However, if it is intended to extract second permanent molars as part of orthodontic treatment, the presence of third molars of adequate size and in favourable positions must be confirmed. It should be remembered that the time of formation of third molars is very variable: frequently they are visible on radiographs at 8 years of age, but occasionally they may not start to develop until 14 years.

Upper lateral incisors. The absence of these teeth presents an aesthetic problem. Sometimes in a crowded arch the canine will erupt in approximal contact with the central incisor and it may be reasonable to accept this position, merely reshaping the canine and building it up with composite as appropriate. More commonly, the canine will erupt close to but not in contact with the central incisor. A decision has to be made whether to close the space (which is functionally preferable) or whether to open it up for a prosthetic replacement of the lateral incisor (which may be aesthetically superior).

Closure of the space is indicated where there is crowding, or a Class II problem that might otherwise require tooth loss for its correction. The angulation of the canine may also influence management decisions – distally tipped canines can be more easily moved mesially.

Space opening is indicated where there is a Class I uncrowded mouth or Class III with little maxillary arch crowding. The colour and morphology of the canine may also influence the treatment decision for aesthetic reasons, and the orthodontist is sometimes called upon to make a decision on future management before this tooth has erupted. Unless the way forward is absolutely clear, it may be better to keep the lateral incisor space temporarily until such time as firm management decisions can be taken.

In summary, the decision to open or close space must be made together with the patient and, where appropriate, the parent after full discussion, preferably involving a joint consultation with a restorative colleague.

Second premolars. It is important that the absence of second premolars should be recognized as early as possible. However, the time of calcification is variable and in a few cases they may not

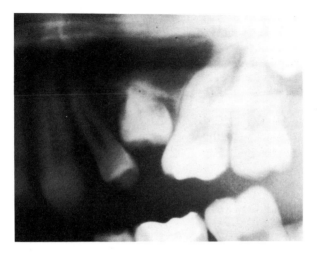

Figure 6.1 A submerging second deciduous molar. Note that the second premolar is absent

become visible on radiographs until 7 years of age. It is essential always to check that second premolars are present before other teeth are extracted for orthodontic reasons.

Where there is crowding or an overjet has to be reduced, the space provided by the absence of the second premolars should be utilized. Where there is no crowding it is usually best to try to retain the second deciduous molars for as long as possible: they may be retained until the patient is 30 or 40 years of age. When they are shed the space will not normally close and, unless there are unopposed teeth in the other arch, little occlusal change may follow. Ideally a bridge should be fitted.

In some cases where a second premolar is missing the second deciduous molar may submerge (Figure 6.1). In the growing patient with a developing occlusion this may lead to quite severe drifting of the first permanent molar. The most satisfactory treatment in these cases is to close the gap, using a fixed appliance to bring forward the permanent molar following removal of the submerged molar.

Early loss of deciduous teeth

The effects of early loss depend on a number of factors including: (a) the tooth lost, (b) the age of loss, (c) crowding.

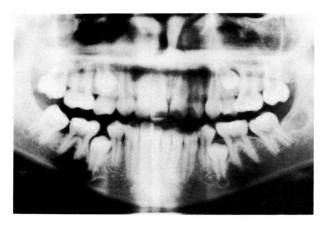

Figure 6.2 A dental panoramic tomograph (see Chapter 17) which shows how early loss of deciduous molars has allowed the first permanent molars to drift forwards, encroaching on the space for the second premolars

The tooth lost

Deciduous incisors. Except in very crowded cases, early loss of carious deciduous incisors has little effect on the development of the occlusion. Where crowding is severe, space closure may occur but space maintenance is not indicated in the caries-prone mouth. If a deciduous incisor is intruded by a blow, displacement or dilaceration of the successor may result .

Deciduous canines. The early loss of these teeth is followed by a space loss as a result of alignment of crowded permanent incisors. The buccal segments may drift forwards by a small amount. Early loss of a deciduous canine, particularly in the lower arch, may result from resorption of its root by a crowded permanent lateral incisor. This is often unilateral and so the crowded incisors will drift to the side of loss with a shift of midline. This is the most serious result of early loss of a deciduous canine because it produces an asymmetrical occlusion which can be difficult to treat unless the midline is corrected. In order to avoid these complications it is good practice to balance the early loss of one deciduous canine by extracting the other deciduous canine from that arch.

Deciduous molars. Loss of contact areas due to caries may produce effects similar to early loss of deciduous teeth. The major effect of early loss of a second deciduous molar is that it allows forward movement of the first permanent molar, which encroaches on space for the premolars (Figure 6.2). Space loss is usually more severe in the upper arch.

Early loss of a first deciduous molar also results in loss of space for the premolars, partly through forward drift of the posterior teeth as in the case of the second deciduous molar and partly as a result of relief of incisor crowding as in the case of the deciduous canine. The space loss from forward drift of the buccal segment is not usually marked, but if the loss is unilateral the centre line will shift to that side. For this reason, as with deciduous canines, it is wise to balance the loss of one first deciduous molar by the extraction of the other from that arch at the same time. This is usually preferable to fitting a space maintainer for the reasons discussed below.

The age of loss
In general, the earlier the deciduous tooth is lost the more severe the space loss will be and there will be delayed eruption of the underlying permanent tooth.

Crowding
This is of major importance in determining the effects of early loss of deciduous teeth. If the arch is spaced the effects of early loss are minor, whereas if there is crowding space loss may be severe.

Treatment
Where possible, carious deciduous molars, second molars in particular, should be adequately restored. However, where one first deciduous molar or a deciduous canine is lost, the simplest treatment is to balance this by extraction of the corresponding tooth on the opposite side of that arch. This will prevent a shift of midline which is often one of the greatest long-term problems following early loss of such a tooth. Balancing extraction for the loss of a second deciduous molar is not usually indicated, but where a second deciduous molar is lost from an otherwise good mouth, a space maintainer should be considered.

Space maintainers. These may be of the removable or fixed variety (Figure 6.3). There are a number of problems associated with the use of space maintainers, including the danger of increased food stagnation and lack of patient co-operation, and so they should be fitted only in selected cases where they will be of positive benefit to the patient. Their use should be confined to the good, dentally aware patient who has lost one or perhaps two deciduous molars and where it is felt that

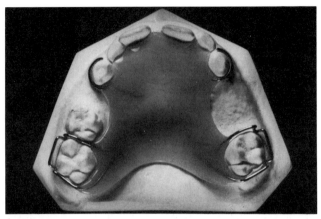

a

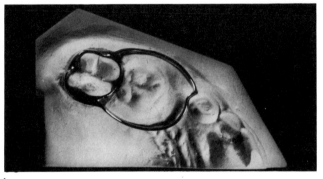

b

Figure 6.3 a, A removable space maintainer. b, A simple fixed space maintainer

orthodontic treatment might be avoided or considerably simpli-
fied by the prevention of space loss. Thus space maintainers are
not indicated for the patient with spacing (where space loss will
not occur anyway), or with moderate crowding (when extraction
of permanent teeth and orthodontic treatment will be needed).
Where it is estimated that there is just sufficient room for all the
permanent teeth or, in the severely crowded case, where the
extraction of one permanent tooth from each quadrant will
provide just enough space, space maintainers may offer definite
advantages.

Loss of permanent teeth

The permanent teeth most commonly extracted because of caries
are first molars, whereas upper incisors may be lost due to trauma.
Both situations present major orthodontic problems. Third
permanent molars are frequently extracted for less obvious
reasons.

Third permanent molars

Some clinicians request the extraction of these teeth as an interceptive measure to prevent the development or deterioration of
lower incisor malalignment in the late teens or early twenties. The
role of third molars in the aetiology of this condition is controversial, as crowding may still occur in patients with congenital
absence of these teeth, and late lower incisor imbrication may
continue to worsen in spite of the removal of the third molars.

Upper incisors

Loss of these teeth is more common where they are prominent,
as in a Class II Division 1 incisor relationship. Following such an
accident, the first concern must be for the general well-being of
the patient and then attempts may be made to save the tooth (if
there has been a fracture) or to reimplant it (if it has been
avulsed). Should these measures fail, an orthodontic treatment
plan has to be formulated. The basic choice lies between utilization of the space (to relieve crowding or reduce an overjet) or
maintenance of the space for a prosthesis. A positive policy must
be followed and teeth adjacent to the gap should not be allowed
to drift in an uncontrolled fashion. This would produce an
unsightly, partially closed space which is difficult to deal with.
Thus unless controlled space closure with an orthodontic appliance is to be undertaken, a single-tooth denture should be fitted
as a space maintainer (Figure 6.4). (It may be mentioned that
where an upper incisor has been fractured, contact areas should
be restored as soon as possible to prevent uncontrolled drift.)
  Usually the best aesthetic result is obtained by fitting a prosthesis to replace the missing incisor and treating the coexisting malocclusion on its merits. This may involve extraction of other teeth.
Sometimes the space of the missing incisor may be used to relieve
crowding or reduce an overjet. To obtain an acceptable appearance it is then usually necessary to crown the lateral incisor on
the side of loss to simulate a central incisor. This is not a simple
solution to the problem since it is often necessary to move bodily
the incisors adjacent to the space with a fixed appliance, and it is

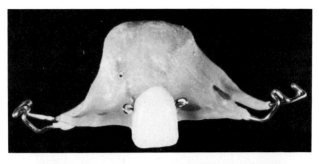

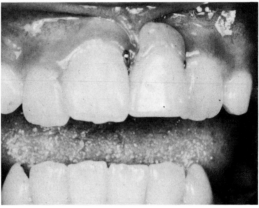

Figure 6.4 A single-tooth denture as a space maintainer. Note the spurs in contact with the teeth on either side of the gap. These ensure that there will be no space loss

not easy to make a good conversion crown if the lateral incisor is small. An additional problem may be the colour and shape of the neighbouring permanent canine. However, in suitable cases it may be worth closing the space as described to avoid the need for a denture or bridge. It is important that a restorative opinion is sought prior to undertaking any orthodontic treatment.

First permanent molars
These are rarely the teeth of choice for orthodontic extraction. However, if their condition is poor they may have to be removed and the space utilized for orthodontic treatment. The timing of extraction is important: early loss in the mixed dentition usually produces superior results to loss in the late mixed or early

permanent dentition. The result of extraction varies between the upper and lower arches, with poorer spontaneous space closure occurring in the lower arch. Before extracting healthy premolar teeth to correct a malocclusion, it is important that the long-term prognosis of the first permanent molar be fully assessed. Unfortunately occasions will arise when, to render a child pain free, the only reasonable course of action is to extract a first molar. The timing of the tooth loss may be less than ideal from an orthodontic point of view. Under these circumstances each case must be assessed on its merits, bearing in mind the guidelines given below, the child's chronological and dental age, the condition of other teeth, the site and extent of crowding, and the willingness of the patient and/or parent to embark on what may be an extensive course of orthodontic treatment in the future. A poorly motivated patient is best left with as many standing teeth as possible (compatible with dental health), rather than removal of additional healthy teeth as part of an orthodontic treatment plan which has no reasonable chance of reaching completion.

Extraction in the mixed dentition (with no active orthodontic treatment)
THE LOWER ARCH. If a first permanent molar is extracted before the eruption of the second premolar and second permanent molar, space closure will occur partly as a result of the forward eruption

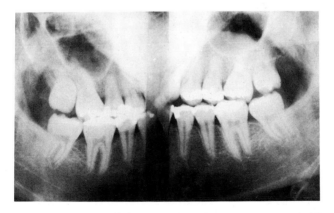

Figure 6.5 The first permanent molars were extracted at the optimal time, just as root formation of the second permanent molars was beginning. The second molars have established a good contact relationship with the second premolars and space has been provided for eruption of the third molars

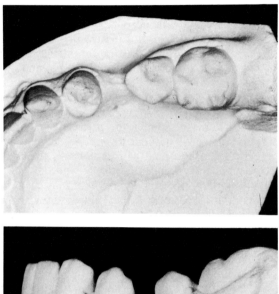

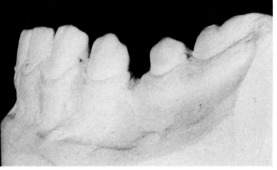

Figure 6.6 The second premolar has drifted distally
following early loss of the first permanent molar

of the second molar and partly through distal drift of the second
premolar (Figure 6.5). This will relieve crowding in the premolar
and canine region and mild or moderate incisor crowding will also
improve. If the extraction is unilateral the centre line will drift to
that side, producing an asymmetric malocclusion. The contact
between the second premolar and second permanent molar is
rarely ideal, because the teeth tip towards one another, but it is
usually reasonable. Sometimes the lower second premolar will
drift distally to a marked extent, leaving a space distal to the first
premolar (Figure 6.6). While this is not an ideal occlusal arrangement, it is usually functionally acceptable and the space is large
enough to avoid food packing.

THE UPPER ARCH. The major part of the extraction space is closed through forward drift of the second permanent molar. If the premolars are crowded due to previous forward drift of the first permanent molar, following early loss of a deciduous molar, this will be relieved. A certain amount of improvement in incisor crowding may follow but this is variable and is less than in the lower arch. Frequently, the second permanent molar will be mesiopalatally rotated but the contact relationship with the second premolar is fair. If the space from the loss of the first permanent molar will be required later to correct a Class II problem, the molar should be stabilized until orthodontic treatment is ready to start.

Treatment planning in the mixed dentition for the patient with enforced loss of the first permanent molars. It is emphasized that the rules for balancing extraction of first permanent molars discussed below apply only in the mixed dentition and where there is no spacing. In the permanent dentition, balancing extraction should not be performed unless the space is required for appliance treatment; in the mixed dentition, balancing extraction should be carried out particularly where subsequent appliance treatment is contraindicated.

The following discussion is based upon the condition that all other permanent teeth (except perhaps third molars) are present, sound and in favourable positions. If this is not so, the treatment plan will have to be modified accordingly.

The best time for extraction of the first permanent molar is just after root formation of the second permanent molar has begun. This is usually between the ages of 8½ and 10½ years. The timing is more critical in the lower than in the upper arch.

CLASS I MALOCCLUSIONS. In the lower arch, if one first permanent molar is in poor condition both should be removed at the optimal time. This will allow maximal relief of crowding and a fair contact relationship between the second premolar and the second permanent molar. The balancing extraction of the other first molar preserves the symmetry of the arch, relieves crowding on the other side and removes a tooth which may well also be cariously involved. If the upper arch is mildly crowded and particularly where there has been forward drift of the permanent molars, extraction of both upper first permanent molars, at the same time as the lowers is indicated. However, if the upper arch is very crowded and if the upper first permanent molars are sound, it is preferable not to extract them but at a later stage to remove teeth nearer the site of crowding (for example, first premolars).

If one upper first permanent molar has to be extracted, the other should be removed at the same time to preserve symmetry but compensating extractions should not be undertaken in the lower arch. Should the upper arch crowding not resolve spontaneously, retraction of the upper buccal segments using extra-oral traction will be necessary.

Sometimes it is suggested that in crowded cases the first permanent molars should be retained until the second permanent molars erupt. These latter teeth can then be held back while appliances are used to retract teeth anterior to the extraction space. In the lower arch a fixed appliance is required; in the upper a removable appliance may be used but treatment is prolonged and the results are often poor.

Occasionally, if crowding is very severe, it is necessary to extract two teeth from each quadrant. In these cases the first permanent molars should be extracted early following the guidelines indicated above and when the permanent canines have emerged into the mouth, the first premolars are extracted. It must be emphasized that these cases requiring the removal of two teeth from each quadrant are rare, and if there is any doubt premolars should not be extracted but the residual crowding accepted.

CLASS II MALOCCLUSIONS. As far as the extraction of first permanent molars is concerned, the two divisions of Class II can be considered together. If a lower first permanent molar is grossly carious at an early age, both lower first molars should be extracted at the optimal time, but compensating extractions of first molars from the upper arch are not indicated unless they have a poor prognosis. The upper arch can then be treated on its merits, usually with extraction of first premolars at the appropriate time.

If the upper first permanent molars are unlikely to remain symptom free until the patient reaches the age to start active orthodontic treatment, it is usually best to extract them early and then treat the upper arch on its merits: the occlusion may be accepted or, where space requirements are slight, the upper buccal segments may be retracted using headgear; but if considerable space is necessary, upper first premolars may be removed and the overjet reduced.

As in crowded Class I cases, the practice of patching up first permanent molars until second molars have erupted and then moving back premolars into the extraction space, commits the patient to a long and unsatisfactory treatment procedure. This may be unavoidable where the poor prognosis of the first molars is not apparent until the early permanent dentition. However, if first permanent molars are removed early, spontaneous improvements of the crowding (but not of overjet) may take place. If subsequently the patient should prove to be unsuitable for orthodontic treatment, it is not necessary to proceed to further active intervention. If treatment is indicated, the retraction of the buccal segments with extra-oral traction is simpler and gives a better result than the individual tipping of premolars.

CLASS III MALOCCLUSIONS. In general, if one first permanent molar is carious it should be extracted early and, provided that the arch is crowded, a balancing extraction of the first molar from the opposite side should be undertaken. Thus if one lower first permanent molar is of poor life expectancy, both lower first molars should be extracted and the upper arch treated on its merits. Equally if one upper first permanent molar has to be extracted early, the other should be removed at the same time and lower arch treatment planned, as discussed in Chapter 12.

Prevention

If one or more first permanent molars are lost early due to their poor long-term prognosis, it should always be remembered that the child is probably in the high caries risk group. In such a situation, in addition to orthodontic considerations, the main responsibility of the clinician is to try to prevent further unwanted tooth loss by employing the full panoply of preventive measures to the remaining teeth.

Extraction in the permanent dentition

THE LOWER ARCH. With no active orthodontic treatment, the effects of extractions of the first permanent molar after the second permanent molar has erupted are often disastrous: the second molar will tip forward and roll lingually; a very poor contact may be established with the second premolar (Figure 6.7) and often a stagnation area is produced; secondary changes in the upper arch often follow producing occlusal disharmonies and plunger cusp mechanisms. There will be little spontaneous improvement in incisor crowding. These effects are particularly marked where the extraction has been performed while the patient is still growing. In the adult, drift of the second molar is less marked and the result is often less harmful, although unopposed upper teeth may over-erupt.

THE UPPER ARCH. Spontaneous space closure is better than in the lower arch and it occurs largely through mesial tipping and mesiopalatal rotation of the upper second molar around its palatal root.

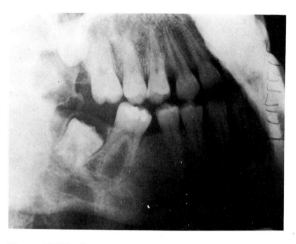

Figure 6.7 The first permanent molars were extracted after the second permanent molars had erupted. Particularly in the lower arch the result is poor

Retained deciduous teeth

The time of shedding of deciduous teeth is quite variable. However, prolonged retention of a deciduous tooth may deflect the successor or prevent it from erupting. On the other hand, a deciduous tooth may be retained due to absence or misplacement of its successor. Unilateral retention of a deciduous tooth is easy to diagnose, but bilateral retention is more difficult. A judgement must be made as to whether this reflects slow dental development or a genuine tooth retention problem.

Incisors
The roots of a deciduous incisor may fail to resorb if there is a peri-apical granuloma, but sometimes the reasons are obscure. Usually the permanent incisor will be deflected lingually as it develops on the lingual aspect of the roots of the deciduous predecessor (see Figure 4.2b). Provided that the deciduous tooth is extracted before the permanent incisor reaches the occlusal level, spontaneous alignment can be expected. However, if an upper incisor (usually a central) is deflected so that it erupts into lingual occlusion with the lowers, appliance treatment to move it labially will be required.

Canines
These may be retained due to malposition of the successor. If the permanent canine cannot be moved into the line of the arch, it may be appropriate to retain the deciduous tooth. It may remain in place for several years if the root and crown remain healthy and it is not subjected to heavy occlusal loading.

Molars
These teeth may be retained due to absence of their successors. However, retained roots can deflect the premolar. If a retained deciduous molar prevents the successor from erupting or deflects it, the deciduous molar should be extracted. Sometimes a retained deciduous molar will submerge.

Submerging deciduous molars (Figure 6.1)
The lower second deciduous molars are most frequently involved and there may or may not be a successor. Submergence seems to be due to ankylosis of the roots with the alveolar bone. As the face grows, the adjacent teeth and alveolar bone continue to grow occlusally, leaving behind the ankylosed tooth which drops below the occlusal level and appears to become submerged. In the majority of cases, the ankylosis becomes resorbed before the submergence is marked and the tooth is shed normally. However, some teeth continue to submerge and become covered by alveolar mucosa. The adjacent teeth will tilt over the retained deciduous molar and quite a severe occlusal disharmony may result (see Figure 6.1). If a deciduous tooth is seen to be submerging, it is wise to keep it under observation to see whether it will become free and re-erupt to reach the occlusal level. If this does not happen and the submergence becomes more severe, the tooth should be carefully extracted. This may not be easy if the ankylosis is extensive. If there is no successor, appliance treatment to close the space may be necessary, and the over-erupted opposing tooth may also require treatment.

Supernumerary teeth

Supernumerary teeth may be found in any region of the arch, but they are particularly common adjacent to the upper midline (Figure 6.8). Such a tooth, which is usually conical or tuberculate, is called a 'mesiodens'. Extra teeth may be found elsewhere in the mouth and may resemble teeth of the normal series. For example, extra teeth in the lateral incisor region may look like normal lateral incisors and occasionally an extra premolar is found. Such teeth,

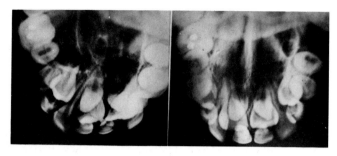

Figure 6.8 Two radiographs showing the parallax method of determining the positions of two supernumerary teeth. The X-ray source of the machine (tube) was moved a few centimetres between exposures. The supernumerary teeth appear to have moved in the same direction. This means that they are palatal to the roots of the central incisors

resembling those of the normal series and developing where there has been an evolutionary reduction in the number of teeth (namely the lateral incisor and premolar regions), are sometimes known as 'supplemental teeth'. In the molar region an extra peg-shaped tooth (sometimes known as a 'para-molar') may be found. It is usually buccal to a permanent molar and may be fused with it to give an extra buccal cusp. Occasionally a fourth molar may be present.

Patients with clefts of the lip and palate have a high prevalence of supernumerary teeth adjacent to the cleft (see Chapter 21).

Supernumerary teeth usually cause crowding and they should be extracted. Occasionally, where there is a supplemental lateral incisor, it is difficult to decide which is the tooth of the normal series and so the tooth in the less favourable position should be removed.

Mesiodens
These are quite commonly found (in about 1% of normal children). They may displace the permanent incisor, usually labially or distally, causing a median diastema; they may produce a rotation of the incisor; prevent eruption of the tooth; or they may have no clinical effect. A mesiodens may erupt and can be extracted simply, but many do not and it is necessary, before surgically removing them, to ascertain their relationship with the central incisors.

Investigation. Sometimes there are no clinical signs and the mesiodens is discovered on a radiograph taken for another reason. If the mesiodens is outside the focal trough of an OPT, it will be invisible on this film. A lateral cephalometric radiograph may not reveal its presence as the roots (or crown if an incisor is unerupted) of the central and lateral incisors may obscure the tooth. An intra-oral peri-apical or occlusal film is the only sure way to reveal the presence of such a tooth. If a mesiodens is erupted an intra-oral film should still be taken as there may be further supernumerary teeth in that area which remain unerupted. Rotation, displacement or failure of eruption of one or both central incisors may be due to the presence of a mesiodens.

Treatment. Supernumerary teeth should be extracted except where they are deeply buried, symptom free and no orthodontic movement of adjacent teeth is planned. If both the mesiodens and the central incisor are unerupted, then removal of the mesiodens is unlikely to result in spontaneous eruption of the incisor. Some form of orthodontic traction, either following exposure of part of the crown via an apically repositioned flap, or by gold chain bonded to the crown of the tooth, will be necessary to ensure the correct alignment of the incisor. Treatment should be undertaken as soon as possible to prevent loss of space, and to harness the eruptive potential of the tooth.

For convenience of reference, the causes of median diastema and of failure of eruption of a central incisor are listed below.

Median diastema
1. Physiological spacing (see Chapter 4).
2. Missing or peg-shaped lateral incisors.
3. Generalized spacing of the upper labial segment, possibly associated with proclination of the upper incisors.
4. A supernumerary tooth.
5. Abnormal labial fraenum.
6. Dilaceration of a central incisor (see below).
7. Rarely a median cyst.

Failure of eruption of a central incisor
1. A supernumerary tooth or odontome.
2. Dilacerated tooth.
3. Scar tissue following surgical intervention.
4. Occasionally there will be no obvious cause and surgical exposure may be indicated.

Anomalies in the form and developmental position of teeth

Anomalies of form

Many anomalies of form are developmental: abnormally large teeth, peg-shaped teeth, geminations and *dens-in-dente* may all give rise to local malocclusions. Sometimes it is possible to adjust the form of the tooth (e.g. by veneering or crowning a peg lateral or removing an extra cusp, remembering that there may be an associated pulp horn) but often it will have to be extracted (e.g. a *dens-in-dente* in the upper lateral incisor region). In these cases, the treatment plan is designed either to close the space or to fill it with a prosthesis, possibly in conjunction with an implant.

Dilaceration
This is the deformation of a tooth due to a disturbance during its normal formation as result of which the root is bent. It may occur in an impacted tooth where the root grows against and is deflected by a hard bony plate. For example, the roots of an impacted lower third molar may be deflected by the mandibular canal. Of greater orthodontic importance is the dilaceration of an upper incisor (usually the central) subsequent to the traumatic intrusion of a deciduous incisor most commonly in the 4–5-year-old child. The already-formed portion of the tooth is displaced while the developing root continues to grow in the original direction. Where the dilaceration is only very slight, the tooth may erupt normally. It may be possible to align the crown using orthodontic appliances, provided that the root remains in bone and does not interfere with roots of adjacent teeth. Where dilaceration is severe, the tooth may fail to erupt. The options are to remove the tooth surgically and maintain or close the space, or to apply orthodontic traction to bring the tooth into the mouth. This decision will depend partially on the degree of dilaceration and the amount of bone available for the root, and is best deferred until the crown morphology can be directly visualized at surgery.

Anomalies of position

Many abnormal tooth positions reflect crowding. However, certain malpositions are developmental in origin: ectopic positions (often involving the upper permanent canine) and transpositions (usually involving either the upper canine and first premolar or lower canine and lateral incisor) must be attributed to abnormal developmental positions. Where the tooth is grossly misplaced, it will usually have to be extracted. Less severe malpositions frequently require fixed appliances to deal with them.

Maxillary canines
Upper permanent canines are among the most frequently malpositioned teeth occurring in approximately 2.5% of the population.

By the age of 8–10 years they should be palpable buccally just distal to the root of the lateral incisor around its apical third. When this is not the case parallax radiographs should be taken to locate these teeth (Figure 6.8). The majority (90% or more) of canines in Caucasians impact palatally, and of these a proportion will cause resorption of the root of the adjacent lateral incisor. If undiagnosed, they may go on to affect the central incisor. Under these circumstances the resorbed tooth should be removed and efforts made to bring the canine into the dental arch. If there are no signs of resorption the choices for management are as follows:

- *Leave.* This is only suitable if the canine is grossly displaced, symptom free, and no orthodontic tooth movement of adjacent teeth is planned. They should be radiographed at regular intervals to screen for pathological changes.
- *Extract.* This assumes that the patient is happy to accept all other occlusal features, often including a retained deciduous canine.
- *Surgical repositioning.* Adequate space and alveolar bone are necessary for this approach. The risk of subsequent root resorption and tooth loss must be fully understood by the patient.
- *Orthodontic alignment.* This is the treatment of choice as it will bring the canine into the mouth with an intact periodontium. The treatment is often lengthy, involving fixed appliances which may be unacceptable to a patient in their mid-teens. Orthodontics will have to follow a surgical procedure which will either expose the crown (if superficial) or lift a flap for the bonding of gold chain to the crown of the tooth. This latter procedure is necessary if the tooth is grossly displaced, or is closely impacted to an adjacent tooth and straightforward exposure would jeopardize the periodontal support of the adjacent tooth. Orthodontic alignment may of course follow extraction of the canine as part of an overall treatment plan to deal with other occlusal problems.

Maxillary first permanent molars

These teeth can develop a mesio-angular impaction into the distal of the second deciduous molar. This will often lead to resorption of the distal root of the deciduous tooth which may cause loss of vitality. A mild impaction may be corrected by the placement of an orthodontic separator between the teeth which will allow spontaneous disimpaction. More severe impactions may be dealt with either by distal movement of the permanent molar using either a removable, or fixed, or combination of the two appliances, or by extraction of the deciduous tooth. The latter option will allow the molar to erupt mesially placed and will certainly result in impaction of the underlying second premolar.

Habits and other local factors

Non-nutritive sucking of a digit or dummy is a habit from which young children derive considerable comfort and security, and is a normal activity in the early years of life. Usually the habit ceases spontaneously as the child grows up and no permanent change will be produced. The occlusal features associated with a sucking habit include:

- *Incomplete overbite or occasionally anterior open bite.* If a digit is sucked this will usually be asymmetrical, with the greatest vertical discrepancy on the same side as the sucked digit (Figure 6.9). Dummies may produce symmetrical or asymmetrical change depending on the preferred position of the dummy.
- *Increased overjet.* The angle at which the digit enters the mouth, together with the vigour of the habit, will determine whether the upper incisors will be proclined. The increased overjet may also be due to retroclination of the lower incisors.

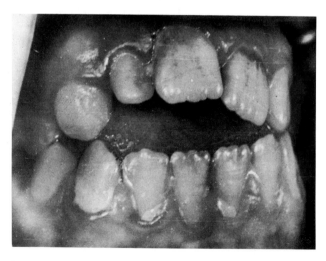

Figure 6.9 A malocclusion associated with sucking the right thumb

• *Narrow maxillary dental arch.* The negative intra-oral pressure developed by the sucking, together with a lowered tongue position and increased buccinator activity will serve to narrow the upper arch with unilateral or occasionally bilateral cross-bite development.

When the child is young, no treatment need be provided. If the habit is vigorous, and persists after the eruption of the permanent incisors, some authorities advocate the prescription of a habit deterrent. This is usually some form of fixed or removable appliance that makes it difficult for the digit to be inserted comfortably in the mouth. If the habit ceases there may be good spontaneous improvement of the dental arrangement. However, if the child has a malocclusion that will require an orthodontic appliance to correct later, it may be better to wait until the start of orthodontic treatment and rely on the presence of the appliance to break the habit.

Upper labial fraenum

In the infant, the upper labial fraenum extends from the inner surface of lip, across the alveolar process to the palatine papilla. When the deciduous incisors erupt, this continuity is normally lost and the fraenum becomes attached to the labial surface of the alveolar process. In a few children the fraenum will persist and this may be associated with a median diastema. Where there is a persistent fraenum, the palatine papilla will blanch if the lip is pulled forwards. It must be emphasized that although a persistent fraenum is often associated with a diastema, it is not a common cause and, in general, treatment should be withheld until the upper canines have erupted to see whether the space will close spontaneously. The causes of median diastema have been listed previously. Occasionally, if the fraenum is abnormally thick and fleshy, it will be a primary aetiological factor in producing a median diastema. In these cases, closure of the diastema and a fraenectomy (see Chapter 18) is indicated, with retention of the space closure provided partly by an orthodontic appliance and partly by the scar tissue resulting from the surgery.

Chapter 7

Tooth–arch disproportion

Disproportion between tooth size and arch size is common. It is usually manifest as crowding but occasionally there is generalized spacing. Tooth size is under direct genetic control, whereas the size of the dental arches depends on skeletal base size and on the soft-tissue morphology and activity: as such the dental arch is both under the influence of environmental and genetic factors. This disparity in the factors influencing tooth and arch size goes some way to explaining the tendency to crowding.

Spacing

This is best accepted unless it gives an unsightly appearance in the upper labial segment. In this region, the spacing may be concentrated in the midline as a median diastema. It is sometimes possible to obtain an acceptable result by moving the upper central incisors together, distributing the space mesial and distal to the lateral incisors prior to a build-up in width of these teeth using composite additions or composite or porcelain veneers. A fraenectomy (see Chapter 18) may then be performed to facilitate complete closure; in addition, this will help to stabilize the result. When a patient first presents with a median diastema it is important to determine if there is a family history: in such a situation there is usually a strong tendency towards at least a partial relapse which appears to be determined by the inherited tooth size. A build-up in the width of the relevant incisors with composite or a porcelain veneer can often be of assistance in such cases since it might avoid the need for long-term fixed retention. Sometimes, if the crowns of the lateral incisors are diminutive and contributing to the local spacing, these may be built up in a similar way.

Where spacing is more generalized and if treatment is indicated, appliances may be used to concentrate the spacing in the buccal segments. Some form of prosthesis (preferably a bridge) will then be required both for aesthetic reasons and to assist in preventing relapse.

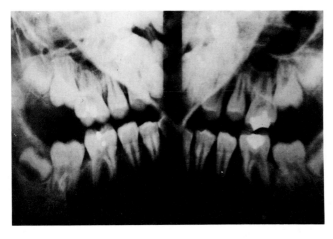

Figure 7.1 Crowding in the upper and lower molar regions. The upper molars are 'stacked'. The lower third molars will be impacted

Crowding

Crowding is common and any teeth may be involved: the incisors and canines if the arch is narrow or short; the molars where the arch is short (Figure 7.1); the premolars and canines if there has been drift of teeth following early loss of deciduous molars (see Figure 6.1).

In general, it is not possible to produce a stable increase in arch size by labial movement of incisors or lateral expansion of buccal segments. Provided that the skeletal bases are long and the molars are not crowded, small amounts of space can sometimes be gained by distal movement of buccal segments using extra-oral traction (see Chapter 15). However, if appreciable amounts of space are required to relieve crowding, extractions are required. Clearly the choice of extraction will be influenced by the poor condition or abnormal form of any teeth. However, in the following discussion it will be assumed, unless explicitly stated otherwise, that all permanent teeth are present and sound. To an extent, the choice of extraction also will be dictated by whether an active appliance is to be employed and the type of appliance. As an example, where crowding of the arches is moderate with little overjet or overbite reduction required, and a fixed appliance is to be fitted, then extraction of second rather than first premolars may be more appropriate. This might save treatment time by reducing the amount of residual extraction space closure required, while also reducing a tendency to any undesired incisor retrusion in a patient with a retrusive lip profile.

Treatment of the upper and lower arches is discussed separately. It is, of course, essential that treatment of the arches should be co-ordinated. This is discussed with the different classes of malocclusion (see Chapters 9–12).

The crowded lower arch

Crowded incisors and canines

Crowding is very common in this area and it tends to become worse with age, in part due to mesial drift of the buccal segments but more importantly due to the uprighting of the lower incisors which occurs during the later stages of facial growth. If the crowding is very mild and the lower arch is not crowded elsewhere, it may be best to accept the irregularity: recent research has shown this area to being prone to long-term relapse, especially where the initial crowding was mild. However, if crowding is appreciable, extractions should be undertaken. Provided that the lower canines are mesially inclined, the extraction of lower first premolars will usually be followed by satisfactory spontaneous alignment of the labial segment. Any residual space will be taken up by forward drift of the buccal segments. Extractions are best undertaken after the lower canines have emerged through the alveolar mucosa but before they have reached the occlusal level. However, the lower canines commonly erupt before the first premolars and so this is not always possible. Should crowding be very severe so that most or all of the extraction space is required, a space maintainer should be fitted. The degree of spontaneous space closure should be assessed approximately 6 months after extraction and where necessary an active appliance prescribed if full closure is a treatment aim.

Where the lower canines are distally inclined, spontaneous resolution of lower incisor crowding will not follow the extraction of first premolars, and lower fixed appliance treatment to retract the canines is usually indicated. Where a lower canine is crowded it is sometimes tempting to extract this tooth. However, the approximal contact between a lower lateral incisor and first premolar is rarely satisfactory due to the shape of the teeth and so extraction of a lower canine should be avoided if at all possible.

Although it often seems to offer a simple solution to lower incisor crowding, normally the extraction of a lower incisor should be avoided for the following reasons:

- Crowding frequently reappears among the remaining three incisors.
- The lower intercanine width decreases and this may lead to a secondary reduction in upper intercanine width with crowding in the upper labial segment.
- It is not possible to fit four upper incisors around three lower incisors: either an increase in overjet or upper incisor crowding may have to be accepted unless the upper canines can be retracted beyond their normal relationship with the lower canines.

However, in a few well-defined cases, listed below, the extraction of a lower incisor may be appropriate, although some of the problems mentioned above still apply:

- Where one lower incisor is completely excluded from the arch and there are satisfactory approximal contacts between the other incisors.
- Where one lower incisor is damaged (e.g. fractured) or where there is extensive periodontal recession so that its long-term survival is in doubt. Fixed appliances are usually required to close the space in such circumstances.
- Where one lower incisor is severely malpositioned so that appliance treatment would present problems. Fixed appliances are still usually necessary to achieve space closure and alignment of the other teeth.
- Where the lower canines are severely distally inclined and the lower incisors are fanned there may be a case for extracting a lower incisor. However, alignment of the remaining incisors requires fixed appliance treatment and it is usually preferable in these cases to extract first premolars and use fixed appliances to retract and upright the canines.

As may be seen, the extraction of a lower incisor is not straight-forward and will often require the addition of a fixed appliance to achieve an acceptable result. On specific occasions it may be appropriate, for example in an adult adjunctive treatment, but it should be remembered that mild crowding of the lower incisors will usually appear better in the long term than any residual dark spaces.

In cases of mild lower incisor crowding, usually when presenting in the adult, enamel stripping, whereby the mesiodistal width of the incisors or canines is reduced, may provide just sufficient space for alignment with a local fixed appliance.

Crowded lower premolars
Where there has been early loss of deciduous molars, space loss may follow so that the premolars are crowded. It will commonly

be the second premolar which is short of space since it usually erupts later than the first. The second premolar may become impacted between the first premolar and first permanent molar or be deflected lingually. If space loss is slight and the second premolar erupts before the second permanent molar, it may force its way into the arch by driving the first molar distally or by forcing the anterior teeth mesially so that incisor crowding increases. Sometimes it is appropriate to fit a lower removable appliance to move the first molar distally. This may be undertaken more readily following extraction of the lower second permanent molar (see below).

In the majority of cases, space loss is moderate and there may also be crowding of the lower incisors. In these circumstances, extraction of the first premolar may be indicated. Extraction of the second premolar does not usually allow a satisfactory spontaneous approximal contact between the first premolar and first permanent molar: the teeth tip towards one another and a stagnation area is created between them unless a fixed appliance is placed.

Where space loss has been severe so that there is already an approximal contact between the first premolar and first permanent molar, the extraction of the second premolar is advised. It should be remembered that the second premolar is slightly wider than the first and so extraction of the latter tooth will not give sufficient space. Severe space loss of the type mentioned above usually follows very early loss of the second deciduous molar, allowing the first permanent molar to erupt too far forward. In these circumstances, the first permanent molar is reasonably upright and an acceptable approximal contact with the first premolar is present.

Crowded lower molars
Impaction of lower first or second permanent molars is rare and probably reflects an abnormal developmental position of the tooth rather than crowding. However, crowding of third molars is very common and, unless other permanent teeth are missing or have been extracted, there is rarely room to accommodate them in the arch. If the lower arch is otherwise regular, the extraction of the crowded third molar itself could appear to be the most suitable treatment. This could be undertaken either by a lateral approach at the time of crown completion or by conventional surgical techniques when about two-thirds of the roots have formed. However, increasingly the limited evidence available suggests that there are few situations where asymptomatic third

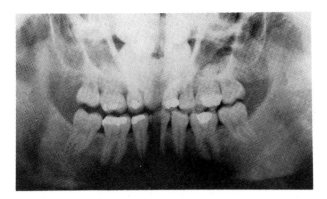

Figure 7.2 In this case, the extraction of second molars has allowed the third molars to erupt into a good position

molars should be removed. No research has clearly demonstrated that impacted third molars are a cause of lower incisor crowding. The contemporary approach to the problem is to consider surgical removal of the third molar if they are causing symptoms or alternatively as part of a definitive treatment, perhaps for lower arch alignment.

Extraction of lower second permanent molars to provide space for crowded third molars is not usually indicated since the position of eruption of the third molar is variable and it will rarely move spontaneously into as good a position as the second molar originally occupied. However, where a small amount of space is also required in the second premolar region or where the second permanent molar is extensively carious, its removal may be indicated. Timing is important. For the best results (Figure 7.2), the second molar should be removed just after root formation of the third molar has started, usually between 12 and 14 years of age. It is important that the third molar is in a favourable position: it should be slightly mesially inclined, its long axis forming an angle of less than 30° to the long axis of the second molar. However, as mentioned above, even when the timing of extraction of the second molar is correct and the starting position of the third molar favourable, it is not possible to guarantee a good result.

First permanent molars are rarely the teeth of choice for orthodontic extraction. However, where one or more of these teeth are extensively carious their removal must be considered. This has been discussed previously in Chapter 6.

The crowded upper arch

Crowded incisors and canines

As in the case of the lower arch and provided that the canines are mesially inclined, extraction of first premolars usually gives the most satisfactory result. For maximum spontaneous improvement of crowding, the first premolars should be extracted after the canines have emerged into the mouth but before they have reached the occlusal level. They should not be retracted with an appliance until they have reached the occlusal level. Care should be taken to ensure that forward drift of the buccal segments does not encroach on the space required for the canines. If space is short, a space maintainer should be fitted.

Sometimes in crowded cases, there is a good approximal contact between the permanent upper lateral incisor and first premolar with the canine completely excluded from the arch. In these cases, extraction of the canine should be considered. The upper canine is slightly wider than the first premolar and extraction of the premolar will not provide sufficient space to accommodate the canine. If the canine is distally inclined or palatally placed and it is possible to obtain a satisfactory contact between the lateral incisor and first premolar by simple orthodontic treatment, extraction of the canine should again be considered. To improve the appearance it may be necessary to grind down the palatal cusp of the first premolar. A problem arises if the buccal surface of the first premolar is distally rotated since the appearance may then be rather poor. In these circumstances fixed appliance treatment may be required, either to align the premolar after extraction of the canine or to align the canine following extraction of the premolar. The treatment of choice depends on the features of the individual case.

If a lateral incisor is crowded into lingual occlusion with the apex palatally displaced and if the canine is erupting in a forward position and is upright or distally inclined, consideration may be given to extraction of the lateral incisor itself. The presence of a canine adjacent to a central incisor does not usually give an ideal appearance and, where possible, it is preferable to extract the first premolar or the canine to provide space for the lateral incisor. However, fixed appliance treatment would be required to move the lateral incisor apex forward. If the patient is unsuitable for or is unwilling to wear fixed appliances, the simple expedient of extracting the lateral incisor may be justified.

Crowded upper premolars

As in the case of the lower arch, it is usually the second premolar which is crowded. If there is a good approximal contact between the first premolar and first permanent molar, the second premolar should be extracted. However, where the first premolar and first permanent molar are not in contact and particularly if there is also incisor or canine crowding, the first premolar should be removed to make space for the alignment of the second premolar. Where crowding is very mild, it may be possible to make space for the crowded second premolar by moving back the first permanent molar with an appliance, possibly following extraction of the second permanent molar (see below).

Crowded upper permanent molars
In the developing dentition, crowding of the upper molars will be manifest as 'stacking' (see Figure 7.1). When they erupt, crowded molars are usually distally and buccally inclined.

Impaction of upper first permanent molars against the second deciduous molars is a result of their abnormal developmental position rather than crowding. First permanent molars are not usually the teeth of choice for orthodontic extraction. Treatment planning, where the extraction of these teeth is necessitated because of their poor life expectancy, is discussed in Chapter 6.

It is usually the third permanent molars which are crowded and if the arch is otherwise well aligned these teeth should be extracted on eruption. If more space is required to allow retraction of the upper buccal segments and provided that third molars are present, of normal size and in favourable positions, upper second molars may be extracted. In contrast with the lower arch, the third molar will usually erupt to obtain a satisfactory contact relationship with the first permanent molar, although on occasions this tooth may rotate around a large palatal root as it descends forwards along the curve of Spee .

Serial extractions

This is a procedure where, in order to encourage the spontaneous alignment of crowded incisors, the timely removal of certain deciduous and permanent teeth is undertaken.

1. The four deciduous canines are removed as the upper permanent lateral incisors are erupting (at about 8 years of age); the alignment of the incisors should improve at the expense of space for the permanent canines.
2. The first deciduous molars are removed in order to encourage the early eruption of the first premolars. This will be most successful if the premolar roots have half formed (at about 9

years of age). It is desirable that the first premolars should erupt in advance of the canines, although this is often not the case in the lower arch.

3. When the upper permanent canines have just emerged through the oral mucosa, the first premolars should be extracted. This is the most important stage of the serial extraction procedure and it is essential to recheck that the case is suitable for treatment by extraction of first premolars: all teeth must be present and sound; the permanent canines must be mesially inclined; and there must be crowding sufficient to justify the extraction of first premolars. If these conditions do not apply the case must be treated on its merits: the fact that serial extractions have been started by removal of deciduous canines does not commit one to going through with this line of treatment.

The full serial extraction procedure has several disadvantages: the child is subjected to extractions on a number of occasions and multiple general anaesthetics are not justified; the lower permanent canine may erupt ahead of the first premolar into the extraction space of the first deciduous molar, impacting the premolar and making its removal difficult; and, quite frequently, the patient requires appliance treatment anyway.

In spite of the disadvantages and limitations of serial extractions as a technique, the principle of timing extractions to take advantage of spontaneous tooth movements is still valid: the removal of deciduous canines under a local anaesthetic to allow spontaneous alignment of crowded incisors may simplify later appliance treatment; and the extraction of a first premolar before a crowded, mesially inclined canine has fully erupted allows it to drift into the line of the arch without appliance treatment. However, the practice of extracting first deciduous molars in order to encourage the eruption of the first premolars should be carefully considered; in certain circumstances it might be valid, but usually such extractions are performed to little purpose.

Arch malrelationships

Arch malrelationships may occur in any plane. Anteroposterior arch malrelationships are the basis of Angle's classification, as have been described earlier in Chapter 5.

Anteroposterior malrelationships

Buccal segments

Anteroposterior malrelationships of the buccal segments often reflect anteroposterior jaw malrelationships but, because the position of the teeth in relation to the skeletal base can vary, it is possible to find cases with normal skeletal relationships and arch malrelationships, and vice versa. When the lower buccal segment is posteriorly positioned relative to the upper, this may be referred to as a Class II buccal segment relationship or as a disto-occlusion; and where the lower buccal segment is forward in relation to the upper, this is a Class III buccal segment relationship or mesio-occlusion.

Labial segments

The labial segment relationship often but not always follows the buccal segment relationship. For example, it is possible to find a case with a Class II incisor relationship but a Class I or even Class III buccal segment relationship.

The aetiology and treatment of the different anteroposterior arch malrelationships are discussed in Chapters 9–12.

Vertical malrelationships

Buccal segments

Vertical malrelationships are not common in the buccal segments.

Where the intermaxillary height is increased and there is a skeletal anterior open bite (Figure 8.1) this may extend into the

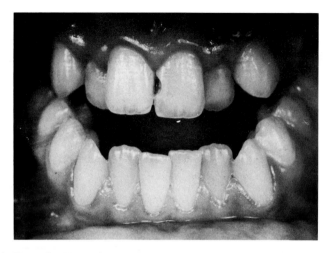

Figure 8.1 This patient has a Class III malocclusion with a skeletal anterior open bite and a bilateral crossbite. These occlusal malrelationships reflect skeletal malrelationships: there is a Class III skeletal pattern; the lower facial third is increased in height; and the maxilla is narrow relative to the mandible

buccal segments, so that perhaps only the most posterior molar teeth are in occlusion. In these cases there is a lateral open bite as well as an anterior open bite. Occasionally a lateral open bite is found in isolation from any other occlusal anomaly. The reasons for this are usually obscure but there may be a localized failure of alveolar development.

Over-eruption of buccal teeth which are unopposed or occlude against a submerging deciduous tooth is of course seen quite commonly.

Labial segments

In normal occlusion the lower incisors occlude with the cingulum plateau of the upper incisors and the overbite is one-third to one-half of the height of the lower incisor crowns.

Increase in overbite
Skeletal factors. It is often stated that a small lower facial height is associated with a deep overbite. However, this is not a constant relationship and occlusal factors (see below) must also play a part.

Occlusal factors. Where there is no incisor contact due to a large overjet (Class II Division 1), the lower incisors will often erupt until they contact the palatal mucosa and the overbite will be deep. Where there is an adaptive anterior oral seal between tongue and lower lip, the overbite is incomplete but is still deep in most cases (see Chapter 3).

Where the overjet is normal and the incisors are retroclined (Class II Division 2), so that the inter-incisor angle is increased, the overbite will also be increased. This may happen developmentally or as a result of an inappropriate treatment of a severe Class II Division 1 incisor relationship with removable appliances so that the upper incisors are over-retroclined. Even if the overbite has been reduced during treatment, it will increase again when appliances are discarded.

The reduction of a deep overbite will be stable only if at the end of treatment the lower incisors occlude with the palatal surfaces of the upper incisors, the inter-incisor angle is within the normal range, and the teeth are in a position of labiolingual balance.

Reduction in overbite

If there is a mild Class III incisor relationship with occlusal contact between the upper and lower incisors, the overbite will be reduced.

An overbite may be reduced and incomplete for a variety of reasons which are dealt with in the following section.

Anterior open bite

Here, there is no occlusal contact between the incisors, and the upper incisors do not overlap the lowers in the vertical plane. Anterior open bite is discussed below according to its aetiology: skeletal, soft tissue, habit and miscellaneous.

Skeletal factors. Where the anterior intermaxillary space is increased, the vertical growth of the labial segments may be insufficient to achieve tooth contact when the posterior teeth are brought into occlusion (Figure 8.1). In the most severe cases only the last standing teeth will meet in occlusion. Generally, the Frankfort mandibular planes angle is increased and frequently, but not always, there is a Class III skeletal pattern.

It is interesting that, except in the most severe cases, the open bite is seldom of concern to the patient either aesthetically or functionally. Frequently, of course, coexisting features such as mandibular protrusion do worry the patient. Correction of the anterior open bite is rarely indicated: orthodontic treatment to elongate the incisors will rarely be successful; extraction or grinding of posterior teeth is definitely contraindicated since the patient will then be forced to overclose into occlusion, exaggerating any prominence of the mandible and possibly giving rise to muscle pain at a later date; overlay dentures are contraindicated because of the problems of food stagnation and because they rarely improve the appearance of this type of patient. The only successful treatment is surgery (see Chapter 19), although such an approach is valid only in highly motivated patients. Of course, if surgery to correct a Class III skeletal pattern is to be undertaken it should be planned to deal with the open bite at the same time.

Soft-tissue factors. Where there is an anterior open bite due to other aetiological factors (e.g. a habit), the tongue will frequently come forwards to fill the gap. This is purely an adaptive pattern of behaviour. A tongue-to-lip anterior oral seal (see Chapter 3) is usually associated with an incomplete overbite. The tongue behaviour will re-adapt on correction of the overbite. In the very rare cases of a primary atypical tongue thrust, the soft-tissue activity is responsible for an incomplete overbite or even an anterior open bite. As discussed in Chapter 3, these cases are difficult to diagnose and may not be suitable for orthodontic treatment.

Habits. Digit or dummy sucking may produce an anterior open bite (see Chapter 6) which will often improve spontaneously on cessation of the habit.

Miscellaneous. The various developmental (e.g. cleft palate), pathological (e.g. bony dysplasia) and traumatic (e.g. bilateral condylar fracture) causes of anterior open bite will not be discussed here.

Transverse malrelationships

Buccal segments

A transverse malrelationship of the buccal segments is termed a 'crossbite' and this may be bilateral (Figure 8.1) or unilateral (Figure 8.2). In most cases of crossbite the upper arch is narrow relative to the lower so that the buccal cusps of the lower teeth overlap the buccal cusps of the uppers. Occasionally, a lingual crossbite or scissors bite is found in which the upper teeth completely overlap the lowers buccally.

Bilateral crossbite

This is a symmetrical transverse arch malrelationship and is usually skeletal in origin. The maxilla is narrow in relation to the

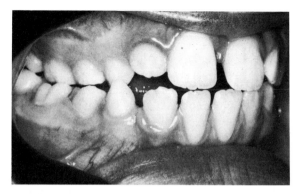

Figure 8.2 A unilateral crossbite. Note that the lower centre line is also off to the right. In centric relation this patient's buccal teeth would meet cusp to cusp, and so there is a lateral displacement to the right in order to obtain maximal occlusion

mandible and this is reflected in the arch widths. Bilateral cross-bites are frequently found in association with severe Class III malocclusions (Figure 8.1), in part because the maxilla is often narrow relative to the mandible and in part because a broader part of the lower arch opposes a narrower part of the upper arch (due to the horizontal discrepancy).

Although, from a theoretical viewpoint, masticatory efficiency is reduced, in practice a bilateral crossbite is seldom of functional significance. Additionally, expansion of the upper arch to correct the crossbite is rarely stable. Thus these malocclusions are usually best left untreated. Occasionally rapid expansion of the mid-palatal suture may be attempted using a fixed appliance. This should be undertaken only as part of a more general treatment plan and although expansion of the suture may be stable, occlusal relapse may still follow.

Unilateral crossbite
It is important to distinguish between unilateral crossbites with lateral displacement and those without.
With displacement (Figure 8.2). In most non-pathological cases of unilateral crossbite, when the mandible is at rest, the arches are symmetrical. However, both arches have the same relative width and with normal hinge closure the cheek teeth would meet cusp to cusp. In order to achieve maximal intercuspation, the mandible

is displaced to one side so that there is an apparently asymmetrical malocclusion. Generally, the midlines of the arches will be coincident at rest, but in occlusion the lower midline will be displaced to the side of the crossbite.

The aetiology of this type of occlusion may be a transverse skeletal discrepancy similar to but less severe than the type causing a bilateral crossbite (i.e. the maxilla may be narrow relative to the mandible and there may be a mild Class III skeletal pattern). However, a unilateral crossbite of this type may be caused by soft-tissue factors. For example, if swallowing habitually takes place without occlusion of the teeth, pressure from the cheeks may equalize the widths of the arches. Similarly with habits such as persistent digit sucking, forces from the cheeks while the teeth are not in occlusion may narrow the maxillary arch so that a unilateral crossbite with mandibular displacement occurs.

The amount of expansion of the upper arch necessary to correct the crossbite is small and, unlike a bilateral crossbite, the occlusion of the teeth will normally prevent relapse. As the maxillary arch is basically symmetrical the expansion should be bilateral.

Without displacement. Here, there is a true asymmetry of one arch which will often reflect an underlying skeletal asymmetry. This may be within normal limits but occasionally it is produced by some pathological factor (e.g. unilateral cleft palate produces a maxillary asymmetry, while unilateral condylar hyperplasia may produce a mandibular asymmetry with secondary occlusal effects).

Clearly, where the crossbite is produced by some pathological factor, treatment considerations will primarily be directed towards the basic anomaly, although occlusal factors are also important (cleft palate is discussed in Chapter 21). A unilateral crossbite without displacement in a normal individual does not usually require treatment but, if treatment is undertaken, it may be unstable.

Chapter 9

Class I malocclusions

This is by far the most common problem, accounting for about half of all malocclusions.

Occlusal and dento-alveolar features

Labial segments

In a Class I incisor relationship, the lower incisor edges should occlude with or lie directly below the cingulum plateau of the upper incisors (Figure 9.1). This relationship need not apply to all the incisors: for example, there may be local irregularities such as rotations or there may be one or two instanding upper incisors. However, taking the labial segments as a whole, there should be a normal anteroposterior relationship between them.

Buccal segments

There may be any type of molar relationship present. This will depend on the teeth that have been lost previously. The buccal segments may be asymmetrical due to earlier asymmetrical tooth loss. This, in turn, may produce a centre-line shift. Because of the order of eruption, if there is a crowded dental arch, the last tooth within the arch to erupt will often be impacted or crowded out of the line of the dental arch. Mandibular second premolars often have a vertical impaction, and maxillary canines are frequently buccally excluded.

Skeletal relationships

Anteroposterior

The skeletal pattern is usually Class I (Figure 9.1), but it is possible to find a Class I malocclusion in association with a Class II or Class III skeletal pattern provided that the inclinations of the

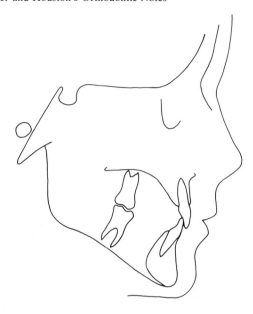

Figure 9.1 A Class I malocclusion associated with a Class I skeletal pattern

teeth, and their positions on the skeletal bases, compensate for the skeletal malrelationship.

Vertical and transverse

The jaw relationships in the vertical and transverse planes are usually within the normal range but there may be malrelationships in these planes and associated occlusal anomalies.

Mandibular positions and paths of closure

Displacement of a single tooth from arch line due to crowding may give rise to a premature contact with the opposing arch and lead to a displacement on closure.

Soft tissues

As in the case of the skeletal relationships, the soft-tissue form and activity are usually within the normal range.

Growth

For Class I malocclusion there will be harmonious growth between the maxilla and mandible which maintains the skeletal relationships in all three planes.

Oral health

As with most malocclusions, except in specific circumstances, a Class I malocclusion *per se* does not pose a specific threat to the long-term dental health of the individual. There are one or two exceptions:

- *Incisor cross-bite.* A lingually placed upper incisor may suffer abrasion on its labial surface from its opposing tooth which, in turn, may be displaced labially with loss of periodontal support.
- *Localized problems.* Partially erupted or impacted teeth, or severely imbricated teeth, may create local stagnation areas where plaque removal is particularly difficult, even for the oral hygiene enthusiast! This can lead to the two major plaque-related diseases of caries and periodontal disease.

Treatment aims

- To improve the aesthetics of the teeth and the function of the teeth and jaws.
- To relieve crowding and produce alignment of the teeth within the arches.
- If necessary, to reduce a deepened overbite and improve the interincisal angle.

Treatment planning

Treatment of the upper and lower arches must be co-ordinated. The general aims of treatment will be relief of crowding and alignment of the teeth. As a rule, it is simplest to plan treatment of the lower arch first, then to build the upper arch around the lower. Usually the size and form of the lower arch must be accepted if the result is to be stable. As a general rule in Class I cases, if extractions are necessary in the lower arch, matching teeth should be extracted from the upper arch. However if there is an asymmetrical problem (e.g. a centre-line shift), then an asymmetrical extraction pattern may be required. Usually the absence of any teeth will necessitate modifications to the treatment plan.

Treatment options

No treatment

The presence of a malocclusion does not automatically mean a need for remedial treatment. Many mild malocclusions can and should be accepted as part of the rich variety of life. Some patients feel that mild tooth displacements lend 'character' to their smile and do not wish treatment.

Extractions

Where teeth are favourably inclined, e.g. mesially-tipped canines, loss of first premolars will create space for the spontaneous uprighting of the canines. Similarly, loss of lower first premolars will relieve the vertical impaction of second premolars and they should then erupt into occlusion. There can be no guarantee that this spontaneous change will occur, and the patient should be reviewed regularly.

Approximately 9 months after the extractions most of the spontaneous change will have taken place and a decision will need to be taken regarding further active treatment (see also Chapter 7 on the management of crowding).

Removable appliances

An upper removable appliance can tip teeth mesiodistally or labiopalatally. Provided that the initial position of the tooth is favourable for tipping, a satisfactory result may be expected. Lower removable appliances are seldom used as they are difficult to fit, constrict the tongue space and have limited space for the active components. Should tooth movement in the lower arch be necessary, a lower fixed appliance should be used.

Single arch fixed appliances

A common approach in the UK is the '2 × 4' single arch fixed, i.e. bands on the molars (the '2') and bonded brackets on the incisors (the '4'). This produces alignment of the anterior teeth

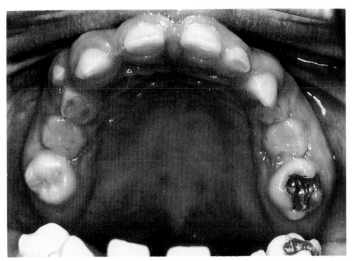

a

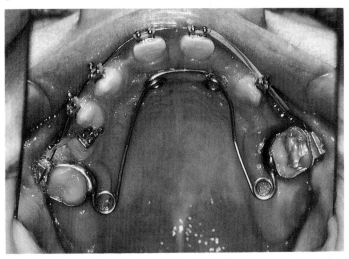

b

Figure 9.2 a, Occlusal view of upper arch of patient with hypodontia. Note that both first permanent molars are rotated mesiopalatally. b, A quad helix appliance has been attached to stainless steel bands on the molars to derotate them, and is now being used to help stabilize these teeth while other work is carried out using a bonded upper fixed appliance

and may be placed on the upper or lower arches. This is particularly useful if there are incisor rotations. A full single arch fixed will clearly give better control of all the teeth.

Upper and lower arch fixed appliances

There is no doubt that this gives the best control of all the teeth and hence a high standard of result. In the severely crowded mouth with anterior and/or posterior rotations, this is the treatment of choice. Adjuncts such as a quad helix may be used to derotate molars (Figure 9.2b), or correct simple crossbites, as well as contributing to molar anchorage. Vertical control of teeth is also possible, elastics being attached to the upper and lower teeth to close down an open bite arising from a dento-alveolar problem such as a prolonged digit-sucking habit.

Functional appliances

Rarely of assistance in the management of true Class I types of case.

Orthognathic surgery

This approach is only of assistance in unusual and specific conditions.

Post-treatment stability

Correction of rotations is one of the major problems of post-treatment stability. Various methods have been tried to enhance stability.

Over-correction. By anticipating the relapse, over-correction of the rotated tooth should allow the tooth to settle in its correct position. It is very difficult to estimate how much over-correction will be necessary.

Pericision. This is severing of the supracrestal periodontal fibres that run between the tooth and the gingivae (see Chapter 18 and Figure 13.2). These fibres are slow to remodel (not being attached to bone), and by cutting through them the tension within the area is released, and new attachments are made with the tooth in its corrected position. This technique has failed to fulfil all its theoretical promise, although the amount of relapse is reduced in teeth which have had pericision.

Positive retention. Using a palatally or lingually bonded retainer, attached to the derotated tooth and its adjacent teeth, there should be little opportunity for rotational relapse to occur.

Long retention. Reitan showed that tension in the periodontal ligament following tooth rotation lasted for about 9 months. This means that full-time retention should last for at least that long. This may be achieved in part by correcting rotations early in treatment.

Combined treatment. Any of the above in combination.

Chapter 10

Class II Division 1 malocclusions

After Class I malocclusion, Class II Division 1 is the most common malocclusion, accounting for about a quarter to a third of all malocclusions.

Occlusal and dento-alveolar features

Labial segments

The lower incisor edges lie posterior to the cingulum plateau of the upper incisors and there is an increased overjet. The overjet may be increased due to:

- Proclined upper incisors as a result of digit sucking, lower lip activity or developmental position.
- Retroclined lower incisors as a result of digit sucking, lower lip activity or, in severe cases with increased overbite, the lower incisors being trapped behind the vertical part of the anterior palate.
- Skeletal Class II relationship. With a severe skeletal Class II relationship the lower incisors may well be proclined beyond their normal angulation, disguising the size of the overjet.
- Any combination of the above.

The overbite is variable and may be influenced by the underlying skeletal pattern or various soft-tissue factors such as tongue thrust or digit sucking. Most commonly, the overbite is increased and complete.

Buccal segments

It is possible to have Class I buccal segments, in which case the upper incisors will be proclined or lowers retroclined. More usually the molars are Class II, with the mesiobuccal cusp of the upper first molar anterior to the mid-buccal groove of the lower first molar.

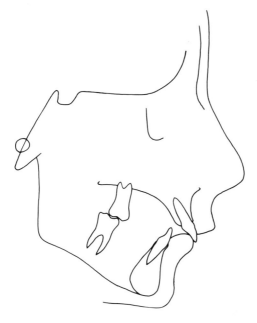

Figure 10.1 A Class II Division 1 malocclusion
associated with a Class II skeletal pattern

Skeletal relationships

Anteroposterior

There is usually a Class II skeletal pattern (Figure 10.1). In many
cases this is the primary aetiological factor responsible for the
Class II arch relationship. The more severe the skeletal malrelationship, the more severe the malocclusion is likely to be and the
poorer the prognosis for orthodontic correction alone. Sometimes,
due to the soft-tissue pattern, the inclination of the lower teeth
will to some extent compensate for the skeletal pattern: the lower
incisors may be proclined and thus the overjet will be less than
might have been expected.

In a number of cases the skeletal pattern is Class I (or rarely
mild Class III). In these cases, it is the position of the teeth on
the skeletal bases that is at fault, due either to their developmental positions or to their inclination under the influence of the
soft tissues or digit-sucking habit.

Vertical

The anterior skeletal face height is usually average, although it may be either high or more rarely low. A high angle or dolichofacial pattern is usually associated with an unfavourable facial profile with little chin prominence. Orthodontic treatment for these patients is difficult. The incisor overbite will often reflect the vertical skeletal arrangement.

Transverse

There are no characteristic transverse malrelationships.

Mandibular positions and paths of closure

In many cases the mandible is habitually in the rest position and there is a centric path of closure. In a few cases the mandible is habitually postured forwards to facilitate the production of a lip seal, the so-called 'Sunday face'. In these cases an upwards and backwards deviation of the mandible on closure will be observed. If there is a well-established postural habit, the patient will be able to close easily into their forward mandibular position, and the unwary practitioner may attempt to correct what, at first sight, appears to be a relatively mild problem. Once treatment has started, the mandibular posture will be revealed and this may present considerable treatment difficulties especially if inappropriate teeth have been extracted. True distal displacements are rare.

Soft tissues and habits

The lips are frequently incompetent (see Figure 3.1c). This often contributes to the lack of control and consequent proclination of the upper incisors. In some cases, a lip seal will be maintained, but frequently there is a tongue-to-lower-lip seal with the lower lip lying behind the upper incisors (Figures 10.2a and 3.2). If, after retraction of the upper incisors, a lip seal will be obtained with the lower lip covering the incisal third of the upper incisor (Figure 10.2b), the outlook for stability is good. If, however, the lower lip does not control the corrected upper incisor position but a tongue-to-lower-lip anterior oral seal continues, the prognosis for treatment stability is poor.

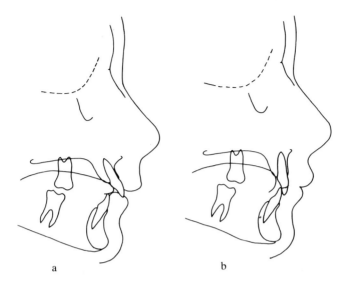

a   b

Figure 10.2 a, An adaptive anterior oral seal with contact between tongue and lower lip. b, Following retraction of the upper incisors, an anterior seal will be obtained by lip contact. The lower lip covers the incisal third of the upper incisors and this will ensure stability of the overjet reduction

In a very few patients, there is a primary atypical swallowing behaviour (see Chapter 3). This will be an aetiological factor in producing the incisor malrelationship and will preclude a stable reduction of the overjet. In these cases the overjet should be accepted.

Those patients with a reduced face height (brachyfacial) will have an everted lower lip resting on the palatal of the upper incisors, and will frequently have a strong mentalis muscle activity maintaining an oral seal (Figure 3.1d). These can be difficult to treat as the lower lip resists the lingual movement of the upper incisors (Figure 3.2).

There is often a history of thumb sucking and in some cases this may have contributed to the incisor malrelationship (see Chapter 6).

Growth

The differential growth rate of the two jaws is generally helpful in Class II Division 1 cases as mandibular growth will tend to

reduce the severity of the problem. Those patients with dolichofacial patterns (Figure 3.1b) will have less favourable growth direction than the brachyfacial pattern, the former exhibiting vertical
mandibular growth, the latter horizontal mandibular growth.

Oral health

An overjet in excess of 6 mm, in conjunction with incompetent lips
in a 7–14-year-old boy signifies a high risk of fracture of the upper
incisors. Unfortunately, unless a functional appliance is prescribed
(see below), the age range over which there is the greatest risk of
trauma is not normally associated with orthodontic treatment.

Incompetent lips are also often associated with hyperplastic
gingivitis around the upper incisors. This is sometimes incorrectly
called 'mouth-breathing gingivitis', although in fact these patients
are not usually mouth breathers (there is often an anterior oral
seal between tongue and lower lip and a posterior seal between
the soft palate and dorsum of the tongue). The gingivitis is a result
of the drying out of the oral mucosa due to the lack of lip cover.
Although in some cases with a deep, complete overbite the lower
incisors occlude directly with the palatal mucosa, trauma is
surprisingly rare.

Treatment aims

- To improve the aesthetics of the teeth and the function of the
  teeth and jaws.
- To relieve crowding and produce alignment of the teeth within
  the dental arches.
- To reduce the overjet but not at the expense of worsening the
  upper lip contour. (Beware over-retracting the upper incisors
  to match a true mandibular arch retrusion.)
- To reduce the overbite and achieve a stable interincisal angle,
  if necessary applying palatal torque to the upper incisors.
- To achieve a good intercuspation between upper and lower
  buccal teeth. This would usually be Class I, but could be Class
  II in an appropriate case.

Treatment planning

The primary objectives of treatment are to relieve crowding and
to correct the incisor relationship. Attention should also be paid

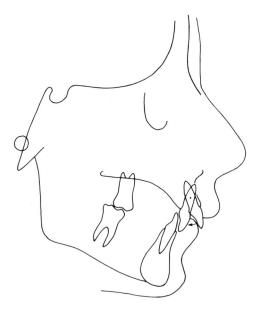

Figure 10.3 When the overjet is large and if the
upper incisors are not sufficiently proclined,
retraction with a removable appliance will produce
a Class II Division 2 incisor relationship

to the buccal segment relationship. In the interests of stability and
occlusal function, there should be a good intercuspation between
the upper and lower teeth. A Class II buccal segment relationship
(which may result if premolar extractions are undertaken only in
the upper arch) is, on occasions, acceptable provided that the
intercuspation is good.

Treatment planning

The lower arch
The lower arch should be planned first. Under most circumstances
the form of the lower arch must be accepted. Proclination of lower
incisors is only acceptable if they are clearly held in a retroclined
position. This means that if there is crowding, teeth usually will
have to be extracted. Space will also be required in the lower arch
in order to level the curve of Spee which is frequently increased
when the overbite is deep. Without extractions, space for lower
arch levelling can only come from such spacing as may already be

present, or arch expansion such as lower incisor proclination or molar retroclination. Transverse expansion is rarely indicated.

The upper arch

The upper arch should be built around the lower arch. If lower extractions are required, then upper extractions will be necessary. Particular attention should be paid to the post-treatment incisor inclination; where tipping of the incisor leads to a retroclined final position, bodily movement and/or torque with a fixed appliance should be planned for and the necessary anchorage requirements considered in the initial plan. A Class II Division 1 incisor relationship should never be converted to a Class II Division 2 pattern by treatment (Figure 10.3).

Treatment options

No treatment

A mild Class II Division 1 incisor relationship may be considered quite attractive, and correction of the problem should only be considered if there are clear oral health or psychological reasons.

Extractions only

This is rarely successful. Loss of teeth will relieve crowding, but contributes no benefit to the anteroposterior incisor relationship. In fact, if anything, loss of lower premolars will encourage some mild retroclination of lower incisors which would increase the overjet. On occasions as a compromise, totally excluded buccal teeth may be extracted when no other treatment is planned.

Removable appliances

If the upper incisors are proclined, and the maxillary canines have an increased mesiodistal tip, then removable appliance mechanics should produce a satisfactory result. In the lower arch, if extractions are necessary, increased mesial crown tip of the canines must be present so that these teeth may upright spontaneously into the extraction site. Residual space should close by mesial movement of the posterior teeth. Remember that if lower canines will be moving distally, the amount of distal movement necessary for the upper canines to achieve a Class I relationship will be increased, and this may influence the choice of treatment mechanics.

Typically, treatment of Class II Division 1 using removable appliances will involve the following stages:

- Extraction of $\underline{4/4}$.

  $4/4$
- Upper removable appliance with:
  Adams clasps on the first molars,
  Southend clasp on the incisors,
  Canine retraction springs (these may be buccally or palatally approaching, depending on the labiopalatal position of the canine),
  An anterior biting platform for overbite reduction.
- Once the canines have been moved distally into a Class I relationship with the lower canines, a second appliance for overjet reduction and maintenance of overbite reduction will be needed as follows:
  Adams clasps on molars,
  Soft wire spurs to mesial of 3/3,
  Wire spring (e.g. Roberts retractor) to reduce overjet (for a full range of labial bows suitable for palatal tipping of upper incisors see Adams and Kerr, 1990),
  Anterior biting platform to maintain overbite reduction.
- The acrylic should be trimmed progressively from behind the upper incisors to provide space for their palatal movement. The wire spurs to the canines will have to be removed in the later stages of treatment to allow contact between canine and lateral incisor.
- Once overjet reduction is complete the same appliance with a passive labial bow may be used as a retainer. If it is unsuitable, a third appliance will be necessary. The usual design for a retainer is as follows:
  Adams clasps on first molars,
  Hawley bow.
  This should be worn full time for 4–6 months followed by a period of nocturnal retention.

(See also Chapter 14 for further details on appliance construction and use)

Anchorage control
There is no such thing as a static anchor point unless an implant or ankylosed tooth is used. It is important therefore to be able to assess the amount of anchorage loss that is occurring. There are a variety of ways in which anchorage loss (i.e. in these circumstances unwanted mesial movement of the upper molars) may be judged:

Reduction in canine–molar distance. Progress of distal movement of canines is often recorded by measuring from a reproducible point on the canine, such as the cusp tip, back to another reproducible point on the molar such as the mid-buccal groove. During treatment this distance should reduce and this may be brought about by one of two things: (a) distal movement of the canine, which is desirable treatment progress, or (b) mesial movement of the molar, which is undesirable anchorage loss.

Canine relationship. If the canine is moving distally, and provided that there have been no lower arch extractions, there will be a change in the canine relationship towards Class I. However, if there have been lower arch extractions the lower canines will also be moving distally spontaneously, consequently there may be little or no change in canine relationship for some time and this may mask loss of anchorage control.

Molar relationship. If no lower arch extractions have been carried out, mesial movement of the upper molar will result in a change in the molar relationship. However, if lower extractions were carried out, then mesial movement of the upper molar may go undetected as the lower molars will be able to move mesially also.

Overjet. If the molars move mesially during canine retraction, the baseplate of the appliance, which is attached to the molars via the Adams clasps, will also move mesially. Contact of the baseplate with the palatal of the upper incisors will, in turn, mean that these teeth will be pushed forward with a consequent increase in overjet. This is probably the most reliable means of monitoring anchorage loss. It must be remembered, however, that the presence of an anterior biting platform will rotate the mandible downwards and slightly backwards, and this in itself will produce a small increase in the overjet. The overjet should always be measured with the appliance out of the mouth, and with the mandible in maximum retrusion.

For methods of anchorage reinforcement and control see Chapter 14.

Correction of a Class II Division 1 malocclusion in which there is an increased and complete overbite and proclined lower incisors, as in a significant bimaxillary proclination, should not be attempted using removable appliances. The resolution of forces on the lower incisors from the anterior biting platform will tend to procline these teeth even further, and prevent full overbite reduction (see Figure 14.14). This is an unstable situation and will lead to failure of treatment.

Single arch fixed appliance

The use of a single arch fixed appliance to correct a Class II Division 1 malocclusion can only be attempted where there is no overbite problem, and is indicated where the angulations of the canines are unfavourable for tooth tipping and/or there are incisor rotations. The need for headgear is also increased as intermaxillary anchorage reiforcement is impossible in the absence of a lower appliance.

Upper and lower arch fixed appliances

This treatment has the ability to deliver the highest quality of result. Control of all the teeth in all planes of space is possible, and the opportunity to use intermaxillary traction to reinforce anchorage can often obviate the need for headgear. Use of fixed appliances is indicated where any of the following conditions exist:

- the angulation of the canines is unsuitable for simple tipping
- the upper incisors are already at their correct inclination to the maxillary plane
- there are anterior and/or posterior rotations
- the lower incisors are proclined or retroclined
- the malocclusion is more severe
- controlled space closure of residual space in the extraction site is required
- there is an increased and complete overbite in an adult.

Functional appliances

Use of a functional appliance is appropriate in specific circumstances:

- there must be two well-aligned arches
- there must be average face height/maxillary : mandibular planes angle
- there should be some proclination of the upper incisors, and minimal proclination of the lower incisors
- there should be a noticeable improvement in the facial profile when the patient postures the mandible forwards
- the patient should not yet have entered their adolescent growth spurt
- it must be accepted that further treatment using other forms of mechanics may be necessary.

See Chapter 16 for a full discussion of functional appliances.

Orthognathic surgery

Severe skeletal discrepancies will not allow the usual dento-alveolar camouflage that orthodontic treatment can produce. A combined orthodontic/orthognathic surgical approach is required. This essentially involves alignment of each arch individually to produce correct tooth relationships and inclinations within each arch. The arch relationships are then surgically corrected and some further orthodontic treatment will be required to settle the teeth into a suitable final occlusal arrangement. This requires careful planning by both the orthodontist and the faciomaxillary surgeon for a successful outcome. See Chapter 19 for further details.

Post-treatment stability

The aim of treatment is to bring the upper incisors under control of the lower lip. This usually means that the lower lip should overlap the incisal third of the upper incisor. If this lip control cannot be achieved, some form of permanent retention may be necessary. This may take the form of a Hawley retainer worn on alternate nights, or a bonded lingual retainer attached to the six upper anterior teeth.

Chapter 11

Class II Division 2 malocclusions

Class II Division 2 malocclusions occur in approximately 10% of the population.

Occlusal and dento-alveolar features

According to Angle's classification, in a Class II Division 2 malocclusion the lower arch should be at least one-half cusp width postnormal to the upper and the upper central incisors should be retroclined (see Figure 5.3). The upper lateral incisors may be similarly retroclined, although in other cases, particularly in the presence of crowding, they may be proclined.

Labial segments

The amount of retroclination of the upper central incisors is closely related to the degree of postnormality of the lower arch which is, in turn, related to the severity of the skeletal malrelationship. The upper lateral incisors, when proclined, are typically mesially inclined and mesiolabially rotated (see Figure 5.3). Otherwise they may be retroclined in a line with the central incisors.

The lower labial segment is frequently retroclined, in sympathy with the uppers, a feature which may contribute to lower incisor crowding but also increases the interincisor angle and so has an adverse effect on the depth of overbite. Often the overbite is worsened by a tendency to dento-alveolar vertical excess of both upper and lower labial segments. In such a presentation, typically the lower curve of Spee is increased and the patient may appear to have a 'gummy smile'.

The overjet is usually only slightly increased, the distal position of the lower arch being compensated for by the retroclination of the upper central incisors. In severe cases where there is a marked Class II skeletal pattern, the overjet may be larger. In this type of case the overbite tends to be deep and complete, the depth of overbite depending on the severity of the skeletal malrelationship and the size of the interincisor angle.

In the majority of patients presenting with this malocclusion, the overbite is only mildly or moderately increased, but on occasions it can be very deep with the lower incisors occluding on the palatal mucosa and the upper incisors on the gingivae labial to the lower incisors. Fortunately, for they are very difficult to treat, these severe cases are quite rare. Most Class II Division 2 cases are mild with a deep but not excessive overbite.

Buccal segments

These may be crowded if there has been early loss of deciduous molar teeth with forward drift of the first permanent molars. Lateral or vertical exclusion from the dental arch of the second permanent premolars is not uncommon.

Skeletal relationships

Anteroposterior

The skeletal pattern is usually Class I or mild Class II (Figure 11.1). The profile is frequently well balanced, although tending to a bimaxillary retroclination, with the chin in a good relationship with the rest of the face.

The receding chin so often seen in Class II Division I cases is not common in Class II Division 2. These malocclusions are not usually associated with severe Class II skeletal patterns unless the malocclusion is a result of an inappropriate treatment where the upper incisors in a severe Class II division I case have been tipped back to reduce the overjet (see Figure 10.3). In the patient presenting with a true Class II Division 2 malocclusion with a significant skeletal discrepancy, studies employing lateral cephalograms have found the cause of the discrepancy to be often an increase in the length of the anterior cranial base, leading to a more distal positioning of the glenoid fossa and thus the mandible.

Vertical

The lower facial height is reduced or average. The Frankfort mandibular planes angle is often low, this reading frequently being accentuated by an upward canting of the distal part of the

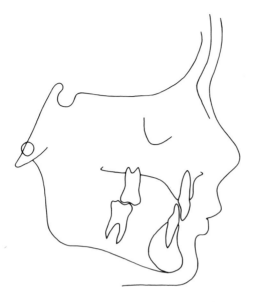

Figure 11.1 A Class II Division 2 malocclusion
associated with a mild Class II skeletal pattern

maxillary plane. The low anterior facial height may contribute to
the depth of overbite.

Transverse

There are no characteristic malrelationships, although in rarer
presentations with a large skeletal discrepancy, a 'scissors bite'
(with upper buccal teeth occluding outside lowers) may be present.

Mandibular positions and paths of closure

In many cases, the habitual position of the mandible is the rest
position and the path of closure into occlusion is a simple hinge
movement. In some of the more severe cases, however, the
mandible is habitually postured downwards and forwards. The
reasons for this are obscure, but it is important to recognize that
the upwards and backwards path of closure in these cases is a
deviation into a position of centric occlusion and is not a distal
displacement. True posterior displacements are sometimes found

in Class II Division 2 cases, particularly where there has been loss of posterior teeth. These patients will often present with pain in early adult life. Attrition facets will be observed on certain teeth. Careful occlusal analysis and equilibration are necessary.

Soft tissues

The lips are held together, usually with minimal circumoral contraction. The lip line is often high, the lower lip covering more than the occlusal half of the upper incisors, a factor which is often important in the aetiology of the condition (see Chapter 3). In some cases there may be an accentuated labiomental fold, and an increased nasiolabial angle with flattening of the upper lip profile is a frequent finding.

Variations in swallowing behaviour are not usually important in the aetiology or treatment of this malocclusion.

Growth

Many patients with this type of malocclusion exhibit a closing growth rotation (see Chapter 2). This will contribute to the reduced facial height and the deep overbite tendency. It may also make the reduction of the overbite more difficult during treatment, necessitating true intrusion of the lower incisors, by means of a fixed appliance, to reduce the curve of Spee.

Tooth morphology

A common finding in this group of patients is a reduced or absent palatal cingulum on the upper incisors. This can be another factor contributing to the excessive overbite. There is also an increased chance of the teeth being smaller than is normal and occasionally a reduced crown/root angulation, although beware the superimposition effect between central and lateral incisors on lateral cephalograms.

Oral health

Oral health is usually good, given appropriate oral hygiene and dental care. In cases with excessive overbite, where the lower incisors occlude with the palatal mucosa and the upper incisors with the gingivae labial to the lower incisors, direct trauma to the gingivae may develop. This often does not arise until the patient reaches adult life and is much more common where there has been loss of posterior teeth. Where inflammation of the palatal mucosa associated with a deep, complete overbite is observed, the symptoms appear to be cyclical. The local oral hygiene is often an important factor in this presentation and should always be addressed first. An excessive overbite is a potentially traumatic relationship; it should where possible be corrected in the early permanent dentition. This is not easy and requires complex fixed appliance treatment.

Treatment aims

* To improve the aesthetics of the teeth and the function of the teeth and jaws, but not at the expense of the lip and facial profile.
* To relieve crowding and produce alignment of the teeth within the arches.
* Where the overbite is excessive, to reduce it. Where the overbite is not excessively deep and there is tooth-to-tooth contact, it may then be best to accept the position of the upper central incisors and concentrate on alignment of the other teeth. If the overbite is to be reduced, the interincisal angle must also be reduced by torquing back the upper incisor apices with a fixed appliance.
* If the overjet is increased, to reduce it.

Treatment planning

It is of course essential to check that all teeth are present, sound and in favourable positions. The absence of third molars will not usually influence treatment unless extraction of second permanent molars is being considered. In fact this approach, or alternatively a non-extraction treatment, is not an uncommon choice in these cases, since space is provided by increasing the arch length when incisor inclinations are changed to improve the interincisal angle.

As is common in other malocclusions, the planning process usually involves an initial assessment of the lower arch to estimate space requirements, especially in relation to crowding, overbite reduction and flattening the curve of Spee. In many cases a bimaxillary retroclination is an integral part of the presenting malocclusion, and for reasons of profile and in the interests of obtaining a good finishing interincisal angle, the incisors may on occasion be proclined. This procedure always carries a risk with regard to long-term stability, but carries the best prognosis in Class II Division 2 malocclusions where incisors often present far more retroclined than normal.

The upper arch is examined from the point of view of crowding, torque requirements (where the upper incisors are significantly retroclined) and anchorage.

Treatment options

No treatment

In milder Class II Division 2 malocclusions in which the typical facial appearance is acceptable, as is the overbite, and the incisors are neither too retroclined nor too crowded, advising no active treatment can be a very reasonable approach to management.

Extractions only

This is rarely an acceptable treatment approach in this type of malocclusion. However, where buccal crowding is severe, with a tendency for the second premolars to be excluded from the arch, their extraction may be an option to consider; always provided that the Class II Division 2 pattern is mild.

Removable appliances

In these types of malocclusion an upper removable appliance is most frequently used to assist in the reduction of the deep overbite during the early stages of a fixed appliance treatment. In a very limited number of cases, a simple removable treatment alone may be appropriate. An example might be where a labial spring is used to tuck a single proclined lateral incisor into the arch. This movement would be performed after an *en masse* appliance (see Chapter 14) had been used to move the teeth of the buccal segments distally in a case where both the incisor alignment and overbite was otherwise acceptable.

The use of an isolated removable appliance, particularly when in combination with a premolar extraction pattern, is rarely prescribed in a Class II Division 2 malocclusion.

Single arch fixed appliances

An upper fixed appliance might be considered where the overbite and upper central incisor inclination is largely acceptable. Extra-oral traction might then be applied to the upper first molars via bands (see Chapter 15). When sufficient space has been achieved by this means or by a second premolar extraction when buccal segment crowding is present, an upper appliance may be fixed to the teeth to align and derotate the upper lateral incisors. Some limited torquing of incisor apices may be possible, as may limited centre-line corrections, otherwise these types of movement are best achieved with a full twin-arched fixed appliance.

Upper and lower arch fixed appliances

The vast majority of patients presenting with a Class II Division 2 malocclusion are best treated through the application of a full upper and lower fixed appliance.

Extraction pattern. The first option always to be considered is whether this malocclusion may be corrected on the basis of no extractions or alternatively loss of the permanent second molars. Often, where the incisors are retroclined, torquing the root apices palatally will increase the arch length and gain sufficient space to both align the dental arches and reduce the overbite. In such a situation a high level of patient compliance is essential, since the result depends on the extra-oral traction (headgear) being worn for long periods to supplement the anchorage. Where the incisors require more torque to achieve an acceptable interincisal angle, there is a deeper initial overbite, or the crowding is more severe, then premolar extractions might be considered (usually four second premolars). Occasionally, when only limited movements of lower teeth are deemed necessary, only upper premolar extractions might be a valid plan in combination with the full fixed appliance. However, if this approach is taken, a Class II molar relationship will result at the conclusion of treatment: there is some evidence that in such a circumstance, especially in Division 2 cases, there is a higher risk of long-term lower incisor imbrication and/or residual spacing in the upper arch since the width of a premolar does not match one-half of a molar.

Overbite. One of the chief reasons for employing a twin arch fixed appliance is to correct the overbite to a stable result. This is achieved by active intrusion of the lower incisors to flatten the curve of Spee. On occasions, an upper removable appliance with an anterior bite plane may assist this process. In the upper arch where there is often an element of dentoalveolar vertical excess, it is also desirable to intrude upper incisors, but this movement is difficult to achieve consistently.

Interincisal angle. In many patients, by definition, this is obtuse at the start of treatment. Obtaining a stable overbite correction is dependent on torquing the incisor root apices palatally to achieve a more acute (reduced) interincisal angle, a solid 'occlusal stop' being formed by the incisor contact. Improving the incisor relationship in this way also improves the aesthetics and function of the finished occlusion.

The full fixed appliance is the most common and reliable approach to the treatment of mild to moderate Class II Division 2 malocclusion.

Functional appliances

Since some functional appliances are most effective in cases where the lower facial height is reduced, their advocates have suggested their use in Class II Division 2 cases. The upper incisors are first proclined to create a Class II Division 1 malocclusion, which is then managed in the conventional manner (see Chapter 16). However, at least initially, the upper incisors are in a position of instability in relation to the lips (outside the area of soft-tissue balance) and the functional appliance must be worn well to hold the upper incisor position while the created overjet is reduced.

Orthognathic surgery

In the more severe forms of this malocclusion where the facial profile is poor and the overbite is very deep and traumatic, a combination of orthodontics and jaw surgery is the best approach. Planning is important (see Chapter 19); however, in an initial phase of fixed appliance orthodontics the upper incisors are proclined to create an overjet while the deep overbite is maintained. The mandible is advanced to reduce this overjet and correct the facial profile. Since the lower curve of Spee is maintained post-surgically there are lateral open bites which are subsequently closed orthodontically by extrusion of lower teeth of the buccal segments to preserve the increase in lower facial height gained in the surgery.

In only a limited number of Class II Division 2 cases is such a combined approach appropriate. Presurgical planning and orthodontics should only be undertaken by the appropriately skilled specialist team.

Post-treatment stability

Lateral incisor alignment
There is a very strong tendency for the lateral incisors to return part of the way towards their original position. This is particularly true if they were rotated. Where possible, the position of these teeth should be over-corrected during treatment. Some authorities recommend prolonged retention, but it is not yet clear whether retention beyond 6 months does improve stability or whether it merely postpones the relapse. As mentioned in Chapter 9, pericision is sometimes performed on these derotated teeth. Correction of these rotations early in any treatment is usually advisable. There is some evidence that these approaches reduce, even if it they do not eliminate, relapse of rotations.

Overbites
As discussed earlier, relapse of overbite reduction will occur unless the interincisor angle has been reduced by palatal movement of the incisor apices. It is sometimes suggested that, in Class II Division 2 cases, proclination of upper and lower incisors (out of muscle balance) followed by permanent retention should be undertaken. The disadvantages of permanent retainers should not be overlooked: removable retainers will encourage food stagnation and plaque formation with consequent deterioration of the patient's oral health, and if they are left out even for a few weeks, relapse will occur; fixed retainers are complex to make and need to be supervised very carefully.

However, there is no doubt that in some patients where there is considerable retroclination of the incisors, the only feasible means of achieving an improved interincisal angle and full overbite correction involves allowing some forward movement of the incisors during the apical torquing process. Such a movement also frequently complements the facial profile. It should be recognized that such movements out of the classic position of muscle balance should be undertaken with caution and the retention phase carefully supervised. Those cases where such a movement of the incisors is likely to remain stable are difficult to select with any degree of certainty.

Chapter 12

Class III malocclusions

Class III malocclusion is found in about 3% of the population.

Occlusal and dento-alveolar features

According to Angle's classification, the lower arch should be at least one-half cusp width too far forward relative to the upper arch (see Figure 5.4). Provided that there is a Class III incisor relationship, the lower incisor tips lying anterior to the palatal cingulum of the upper incisors, milder degrees of prenormality are also included in this group of malocclusions.

Labial segments

The upper incisors are often crowded and they are usually proclined. The lower incisors may be slightly crowded but they are often spaced. Frequently the lower incisors are retroclined. Thus in many cases, the inclination of the incisors compensates to an extent for the underlying sagittal arch malrelationship. In other words, there is usually dento-alveolar compensation of a Class III skeletal pattern.

By definition there is a Class III incisor relationship when the lower incisor edges are lying anterior to the cingulum plateau of the upper incisors. The lower incisors may lie anterior to the uppers so that there is a reverse overjet (see Figure 5.4) and an anterior displacement on closure may have contributed to this. The overbite varies considerably between cases. If there is incisor contact, the overbite will be reduced. Frequently if the anterior intermaxillary height is increased (and there is a large Frankfort- or maxillary–mandibular planes angle), there will be an anterior open bite (see Figure 8.1). Occasionally when there is a reverse overjet and the anterior intermaxillary height is low, the overbite will be deep.

Buccal segments

Frequently the upper arch is short anteroposteriorly so that the buccal segments are crowded: the canines may be mesially inclined and the first permanent molars distally inclined. In the developing occlusion, second and third molars may have become stacked and impacted (see Figure 7.1). Where there has been early loss of deciduous molar teeth, space reduction is rapid in the crowded upper arch. Often the lower arch is long and there may be spacing. A frequent presentation is of a crowded upper arch with canines buccally excluded, while the lower arch is well aligned.

In the vertical plane, if there is an anterior open bite, this may extend into the buccal segments, and in the most severe cases only the last erupted molars meet in occlusion. Not infrequently, there is a crossbite in the buccal segments. This may be unilateral or bilateral. A unilateral crossbite is usually associated with lateral displacement of the mandible to obtain maximal intercuspation (see Chapters 4 and 8).

In the transverse plane, crossbites are often present (see Figure 8.1), in part because the upper arch is narrow relative to the lower and in part because, with the Class III anteroposterior occlusal discrepancy, a wider part of the lower arch opposes a given part of the upper.

Skeletal relationship

The skeletal pattern is frequently the most important factor in producing a Class III malocclusion.

Anteroposterior

Usually there is a Class III skeletal pattern (Figure 12.1). The more adverse the skeletal pattern, the more severe the Class III malocclusion is likely to be and the less amenable to treatment, except by surgery.

Although attention is often focused on a large mandible, it must be remembered that a Class III skeletal pattern is also frequently associated with a short retrognathic maxilla and a forward position of the glenoid fossae on the skull base, so that the mandible is more anteriorly positioned than usual. The anterior cranial base is frequently short.

Rarely is the skeletal malrelationship due to a single anomalous factor. More commonly it is a combination of factors (mandible,

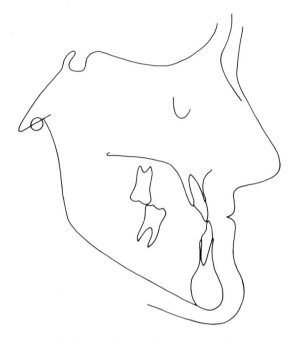

Figure 12.1 A Class III malocclusion associated with a
Class III skeletal pattern

maxilla and cranial base) which, although each may just be within
the normal range, combine to produce an overall Class III skeletal effect.

Although the majority of Class III malocclusions are associated
with a Class III skeletal pattern, it is possible to have a Class III
malocclusion with a Class I skeletal pattern. In these cases the
inclination of the teeth or their positions on the skeletal base are
responsible for the anteroposterior arch malrelationship.

Vertical

Frequently the anterior height of the intermaxillary space is high.
The Frankfort mandibular planes angle is correspondingly high.
This is associated with a reduced overbite or anterior open bite.
However, in some cases the Frankfort mandibular planes angle is
average or even low and the overbite may be normal in amount

or deep (with the lower incisors lying anterior to the uppers). Therefore there is a wide variation in the intermaxillary height and it is important to identify and quantify this variable in the diagnosis since it will greatly affect the treatment plan.

Transverse

In many but not in all cases, the maxillary base is narrow and the mandibular base wide. The resulting transverse discrepancy is aggravated by the forward position of the mandible relative to the maxilla: as in the case of the dental arches, the skeletal bases diverge posteriorly so that when the lower base is in a forward position, a wider part lies below a given part of the maxilla. In many cases, the transverse discrepancy is compensated for by a buccal inclination of the upper teeth and a lingual inclination of the lower teeth. However, if this is not sufficient there will be a crossbite.

Some authors divide patients with Class III malocclusions into two subgroups according to their facial pattern. One subgroup would have a small, narrow maxilla and a mandible of normal length but with a large gonial angle, so that the Frankfort mandibular planes angle is increased. The other subgroup of the Class III skeletal pattern would be due to the large mandible rather than the short maxilla. The Frankfort mandibular planes angle would be either average or low. Although patients corresponding to these types are found, the majority of Class III cases have features of both groups and so this allocation of patients to groups is not satisfactory. It does, however, draw attention to the wide range of facial patterns which may be associated with Class III malocclusions and how these must be recognized in any treatment planning process.

Mandibular positions and paths of closure

Usually there is a simple hinge closure from rest to occlusion. In a number of cases with a mild Class III incisor relationship and a normal or increased overbite, when the mandible is in centric relation, the incisors would meet edge to edge (with the posterior teeth out of occlusion) but, in order to obtain a position of maximal occlusion, there is a forward displacement of the mandible which exaggerates the severity of the occlusal and skeletal base malrelationship or discrepancy. A few of these cases may also overclose.

Where there is a unilateral crossbite with the teeth in occlusion there will usually be an associated lateral displacement of the mandible on closure. In theory, patients with occlusal disharmonies and mandibular displacements of the types described may be more liable to suffer from muscle pain, although there is limited evidence to support this contention. However, since it is straightforward, it usually makes sense to correct such displacements early as a simple interceptive measure. However, where the maxillary base is narrow and the inclination of the teeth already compensates for this to some extent, simple arch expansion may not be stable.

Soft tissues

Where the anterior intermaxillary height is large, the lips are frequently incompetent. Such cases often have a skeletal anterior open bite, and during swallowing there will be an adaptive variation of swallowing behaviour with the tongue coming forwards into the gap between the incisors. Where the intermaxillary height is reduced, sometimes the upper lip may also be shorter and hypotonic.

Growth

In most Class III cases it is usually best to proceed on the basis that any growth will be unfavourable, at least until this assumption is proved wrong! This is due to the fact that dento-alveolar compensation is often at its limit by the time the patient enters the prepubertal growth spurt, the mandible grows more prognathic relative to the maxilla and further dento-alveolar adaptation is not possible.

Where the height of the intermaxillary space is normal or reduced, such growth may result in a worsening of the reverse overjet and the horizontal profile of the face. Where the height of the intermaxillary space is increased with growth, the tendency to a skeletal anterior open bite may become greater as the effect of the opening growth rotation (see Chapter 2) continues. Similarly, the growth tendency, in this case vertical, exceeds the limits of dento-alveolar adaptation and the anterior open bite may dramatically worsen with only posterior molars in contact. In such cases there is often a similarly dramatic effect on the vertical profile of the face.

Oral health

Mandibular displacements due to occlusal disharmonies eventually may be associated with muscle pain, although it should be stressed that this might be only one factor contributing to temporomandibular joint pain dysfunction syndrome. Where there is a premature contact in the incisor region there may be gingival recession around one or more lower incisors, but this is more common in Class I cases with a single instanding upper central incisor and an associated anterior displacement. Although in cases where there is an anterior open bite, periodontal changes might be expected around the nonfunctional teeth (those out of occlusion), no characteristic problems are found.

Treatment aims

- To improve the aesthetics of the teeth and the function of the teeth and jaws while maintaining or improving the facial profile.
- To relieve crowding and produce alignment within the arches.
- To correct the incisor relationship to obtain a more normal overjet, overbite and interincisal angle.
- To eliminate anteroposterior and unilateral lateral crossbites together with associated displacements.

Treatment planning

When treatment planning a Class III case, it is important to establish the true occlusal position after all displacements have been eliminated. It is often of value to have two sets of records – one with the occlusion in the displaced position and the other set at the retruded condylar position with displacements eliminated. The patient will often present complaining of upper arch (canine) crowding associated with a narrow and/or short dental arch. In such cases the crowding should not be relieved without some consideration being given to the likely effect of future growth on the dental arch relationship. It is wise to develop a longer term provisional treatment plan before arranging extraction of any permanent teeth.

Treatment options

No treatment

Where crowding of the dental arches is minimal, there are no displacements apparent and the Class III appearance of the incisors and/or the jaws is acceptable, this is a reasonable approach to management. It also holds certain advantages from the point of view of keeping the Class III growth tendency under review and minimizing any intervention until growth has largely finished and the jaw profile has been finally established.

Extractions only

In many cases where the lower arch is well aligned, the upper arch is crowded, there is no displacement and the appearance of the Class III incisor and jaw discrepancy is acceptable to the patient, upper arch extractions only may appear a simple and attractive treatment. Usually upper first premolar loss is considered to facilitate the alignment of buccally excluded upper permanent canines, always provided that they are favourably (mesially) inclined.

Great care should be taken with this approach, since upper incisors can drop back into any residual extraction space, to worsen the incisor pattern. However, on occasions it is appropriate; although an upper removable space maintainer may, in addition to its usual role, act to support the position of the labial segment.

Removable appliances

Treatment with an upper removable appliance works particularly well where one or two incisors are 'caught behind the bite' and there is an associated forward displacement of the lower jaw. Such an approach is most frequently employed as an interceptive measure in the mixed dentition. An adequate overbite is essential at the completion of tooth movement to maintain the correction.

Occasionally a removable appliance may be used in company with a fixed appliance to clear the occlusion during the early stages of treatment, or alternatively to provide an intermittent anchor in the lower arch from which to attach Class III intermaxillary elastics to an upper fixed appliance.

Single arch fixed appliances

An upper single arch fixed appliance may be considered when the lower is well aligned, the jaw and incisor discrepancy is acceptable to the patient, there is no displacement but there are substantial rotations in the maxillary arch. Depending on the crowding, either first or second premolars would often be extracted.

Full arch fixed appliances

This would be the usual orthodontic approach to a purely dento-alveolar correction of this type of malocclusion. Before prescribing such an appliance, a careful assessment is required. The underlying skeletal discrepancy should be relatively mild and susceptible to dento-alveolar camouflage otherwise surgery will be necessary to achieve a correction. Ideally the upper incisors should at presentation be upright or retroclined and the lowers proclined, such that they may be tipped to make the correction. It is an advantage if there is also an initial anterior displacement on closure. The patient should be checked to see if they can obtain an edge-to-edge incisor contact; this is often indicative of a good prognosis for treatment provided that the incisal inclinations are favourable.

Before starting such treatment, due consideration should be given to the pattern of growth since if this is unfavourable it could rapidly outstrip the amount of dento-alveolar movement available to disguise the underlying horizontal skeletal discrepancy.

In patients with a tendency towards an increased lower facial height, special care should be taken since most tooth movements in this type of case will tend to open the bite on the molars and encourage a further increase in the anterior intermaxillary height. This is especially true when upper arch expansion devices are employed (see Chapter 15). In patients with this type of tendency (towards an anterior open bite), growth modification may be possible by means of a high pull headgear to the upper first permanent molars. Such an approach is very dependant on active growth and good patient co-operation.

Extraction pattern. This will of course depend on the amount of horizontal movement of the incisors required and the degree of crowding present. In a typical case where upper incisors are to be tipped forwards (thus adding space to the arch) and the lower incisors are to be tipped back, a common extraction pattern might be removal of upper second premolars and lower first premolars.

Overbite. It is usually important to finish treatment with a positive overbite in order to maintain the incisor correction.

Interincisal angle. This should be within normal limits at the conclusion of treatment. If upper incisors are proclined too far or the lowers over-retroclined, not only may the result be unstable but the health of the supporting tissues may be prejudiced. In particular, transverse loading of an upper incisor can result in rapid periodontal breakdown.

In a suitable case a full fixed appliance can give an excellent and consistent result. However, case selection is particularly important in Class III cases. If dento-alveolar camouflage is attempted in a patient with a strongly active unfavourable growth pattern, not only will treatment fail but future skeletal correction employing surgery may have been prejudiced also.

Functional appliances

This has been a popular treatment approach in Class III malocclusion in the past, the Fränkel FR 3 (see Chapter 16) being a commonly used appliance. Usually, such an appliance was fitted early in the mixed dentition stage of occlusal development. Problems with the long-term retention of the occlusal result during continuing growth and the essentially dento-alveolar nature of the correction have made such functional appliances less popular in contemporary orthodontic management of Class III malocclusion.

Orthognathic surgery

This has become increasingly popular in the treatment of patients with moderate to severe Class III skeletal discrepancy. An initial orthodontic phase is usually necessary in these patients to decompensate the arches by putting the teeth in the ideal positions to facilitate the surgery. The maxilla may be advanced or the mandible pushed back as the patient's profile and occlusion demands. Often a combination of upper and lower jaw surgery is necessary, with the addition of a reduction genioplasty of the chin.

Vertical skeletal excess may be dealt with by the addition of a Le Fort 1 posterior impaction osteotomy. This is a commonly employed approach to the problem of skeletal anterior open bite.

A more detailed description of surgical correction of Class III malocclusions is given in Chapter 19.

Over the past decade, surgical correction has become a common approach to patients with significant Class III jaw and/or facial profile discrepancies. If a young patient shows early signs of developing such a problem and there is a chance of further unfavourable growth, dento-alveolar camouflage generally should be avoided. Such untimely interventions can create problems later if orthognathic correction is to be considered.

Surgery in these cases would be performed usually when all growth has ceased, since otherwise there is a danger of the skeletal discrepancy regrowing.

Post-treatment stability

Stability of overjet correction depends in the short term on an adequate overbite and in the long term on facial growth. The greater part of orthodontic treatment is undertaken in the growing patient. On average, the mandible grows downwards and forwards slightly faster than the maxilla. In Class III patients this is an adverse growth trend and may result both in a worsening (or relapse) of the overjet and a reduction in overbite. An early sign of this happening is loss of overbite on the upper lateral incisors, with the result that they relapse into a reverse overjet.

In some patients the Class III skeletal pattern will become markedly more severe after treatment and in these cases relapse is inevitable. In other patients the facial proportions change little during the later stages of growth and no adverse occlusal changes should result. In Class III, more than other types of malocclusion, long-term stability depends on a favourable growth pattern and this holds true whatever treatment approach is adopted.

Chapter 13

Tissue changes associated with tooth movement

The arrangement by which a tooth is suspended in a socket in the alveolar bone via the periodontal ligament is well known.

Normal alveolar bone. This consists of a layer of lamellated compact bone adjacent to both the periodontal membrane (lamina dura) and the oral mucosa. Cancellous or spongy bone is found between these two compact layers. The lamellae of the compact bone run parallel to the long axis of the tooth. On the labial or buccal sides of the alveolar crest, the bone is almost entirely compact.

The physical properties of bone situated elsewhere in the body and its reaction to different stresses is relatively well understood. However, this is not necessarily the case when examining those bony changes in the alveolus that occur in relation to stress associated with tooth loading.

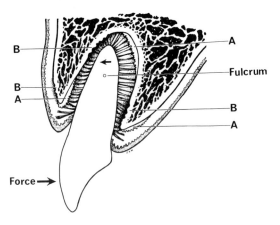

Figure 13.1 The effects of a tipping force: A, areas of bone deposition; B, areas of bone resorption

Periodontal ligament. In general, much less is known of the properties of the periodontal ligament than of those for bone. Histologically, it consists of collagenous connective tissue, cells, blood vessels and tissue fluids; additionally, it would appear to be viscoelastic although, apart from this, the physical properties are poorly defined. However, it would seem that as well as cushioning the tooth against sudden blows, having a role in eruption and mediating sensory response, this ligament is also vital in the process of orthodontic tooth movement.

The classic experiments on tissue changes following orthodontic loading and initial tooth movement were performed by Sandstedt (1901), by Oppenheim, first on monkeys and then on humans (1912, 1933 and 1947), and later by Reitan (1960). Much of our current understanding of tooth movement is still based on these early studies.

Types of tooth movement

Tipping (Figure 13.1)
This is produced typically by application of a single point force via a removable orthodontic appliance. With light forces, the fulcrum is about 40% of the length of the root from the apex.

Bodily movement and rotation
Usually, these are not practicable with removable appliances since they require the application of a force couple. However, most fixed appliances are capable of producing bodily tooth movements and rotations through their potential to transport both crown and root through three dimensions of space.

Extrusion and intrusion
The force distribution within the periodontal ligament depends on the nature of the tooth movement. With tipping movements, areas of maximal pressure and tension are set up at the apical and cervical regions of the root, whereas with bodily movements the force is distributed reasonably evenly along the root axis. Extrusion and intrusion of teeth is also possible, although much reduced forces are required in the latter instance since the force is being concentrated at the small apical area of the root.

Tissue changes

The tissue changes produced depend principally on the values and duration of the forces used. Different regions of the periodontal ligament may show different types of tissue reaction at the one time depending on the force values within the periodontium at that particular point.

Within the first 24 hours after the application of the force, the tooth moves some way through the periodontal space, setting up areas of tension and compression within the periodontium. This initial movement appears to be, at least in part, a viscoelastic effect.

Areas of pressure

Light forces (typically 30 g or approximately 0.3 N per single-rooted tooth for tipping movement). The periodontal ligament is compressed but not crushed and the blood vessels remain patent. Within 24–48 hours, osteoclasts appear along the bone surface and direct bone resorption proceeds. Within the cancellous spaces, deposition of osteoid takes place.

Heavy forces. The periodontal ligament is crushed between the tooth and the socket wall. The blood vessels are occluded and the periodontal ligament becomes acellular and hyaline in appearance. The osteocytes of the underlying bone die. These hyalinized areas are often fairly localized, and adjacent to them and within the cancellous spaces of the underlying bone osteoclasts appear. In this manner the hyalinized area is removed by undermining resorption and the tooth will eventually move. If the range of action of the force (e.g. spring) has been large, the force applied will still be excessive and further areas of hyalinization will appear.

Areas of tension

Initially there is a proliferation of fibroblasts and preosteoblasts and the periodontal fibres are elongated. Osteoid tissue is deposited along the bone surface in spicules, lying in the direction of the stretched periodontal fibres. Subsequently this osteoid tissue is progressively replaced by bundle bone.

Where heavy forces have been used, the periodontal fibres on the tension side may be torn and blood vessels ruptured. When the tooth is being moved labially or palatally, modelling resorption and deposition on the external alveolar surface, particularly in the marginal region, will maintain the thickness and contour of the alveolar plates.

Retention

Retention is the term applied to that period of treatment during which the teeth are held passively after orthodontic correction has

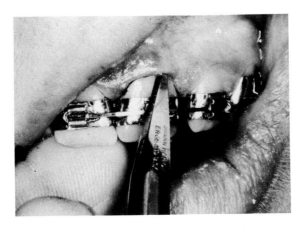

Figure 13.2 Pericision. The free gingival fibres and trans-
septal fibres are severed

been achieved. During the period of retention, further tissue changes take place. In the tension areas the remaining osteoid is replaced by bundle bone which in turn is reorganized to form lamellated bone with Haversian systems.

In the regions of pressure, the osteoclasts remain for up to 2 weeks. Osteoid is deposited over the areas of resorption and, in due course, this is replaced by bundle bone and ultimately by mature lamellated bone.

The periodontal fibres also become reorganized during the retention period. Most of these changes are completed within 6 months. However, reorganization is much slower after certain tooth movements; for example, after rotations, the trans-septal and free (circum) gingival fibres remain displaced for a considerable time. It is possible that the failure of readaptation of these fibres contributes towards relapse of such tooth movements. For this reason, surgical section or pericision (Figure 13.2) of these fibres may be undertaken following tooth alignment. This does not always eliminate relapse but appears to be effective in reducing the relapse tendency provided that it is correctly performed. The tooth should then be retained in the conventional manner for about 6–9 months. Another approach to this problem is to correct any tooth rotations early in the active treatment phase; they are then effectively retained throughout appliance therapy.

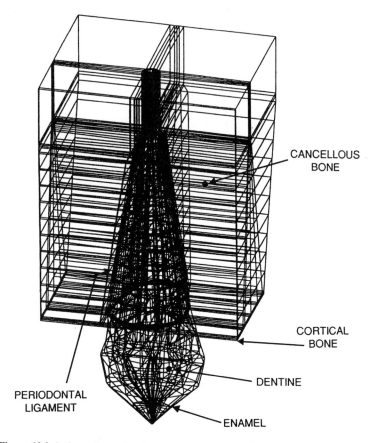

Figure 13.3 A three-dimensional computer model as used to investigate tooth movement

Force and tissue change – the contemporary view.

The preceding description of tissue change in reaction to a force on a tooth was first described nearly 40 years ago. However, the precise mechanism by which stresses are set up within the periodontal ligament and how such stresses mediate cellular change with resultant orthodontic tooth movement is still not understood. Computer models employing sophisticated finite element stress analysis software, as previously applied to bridge

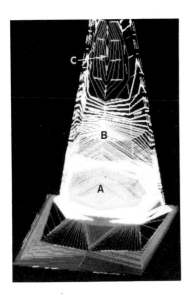

Figure 13.4 To show the complicated pattern of stresses in the periodontal ligament: A, compression; B, intermediate; C, tension. Viewed from the direction the tooth is moving

and building design in engineering, have recently been used to define these stresses together with the resultant strains. Such a three-dimensional model (Figures 13.3 and 13.4) confirms the basic although simplistic description given previously (Figure 13.1), but it also demonstrates that the arrangement of stresses in the ligament is constantly changing both with regard to magnitude and direction. This holds true even in the scenario of a steady single point load applied to a single rooted tooth.

This more recent type of study has also indicated that, although the traditional view of a single rooted tooth tipping about a point 40% from the apex makes sense in a two-dimensional diagram, in the true situation where one is operating in three dimensions the picture is more complicated. The centre of rotation appears to move constantly within an elliptical area towards the apical third of the root (McGuinness *et al.*, 1992).

The factors linking stress to cellular response are also largely unknown although piezoelectric and various chemical factors (for example prostaglandins) have been implicated (Sandy and Harris, 1984).

This lack of detailed knowledge on how teeth move goes some way to explaining the unpredictability of individual tooth response in the clinical situation.

Force magnitude

The threshold value below which tooth movement will not occur is very low. For tipping movements, a very light force should be applied initially and this can be increased to about 30–70 g (0.3–0.7 N) for a single rooted tooth. The force applied should be proportional to the root area and correspondingly heavier forces may be applied to molar teeth.

Heavier forces may also be used for bodily tooth movement, as the force is more evenly distributed throughout the periodontal ligament.

Shown below are possible ranges for force application to a typical single rooted tooth. Larger forces may be appropriate where larger rooted teeth are to be moved, especially when in groups and when applied intermittently (to approximately convert grams to newtons divide by 100).

tip = 30–70 g ; bodily = 100–150 g ; extrude = 30–100 g ; intrude = 10–30 g

The rate of tooth movement

About 1 mm per month may be regarded as an acceptable rate of tooth movement. However, various factors, including the rate of growth and local tissue turnover, may affect the rate of tooth movement.

The nature and duration of the force applied

Both light and heavy forces will result in orthodontic tooth movement. However, it is generally felt that light continuous forces minimize hyalinization of the periodontal ligament, the rate of tooth movement being faster and more efficient. Heavier intermittently applied force is less likely to maintain a physiological tissue response.

The effect of age

In the adult, the periodontal ligament is much less cellular than in the child. In addition, the alveolar bone in children is less dense than in older patients. This means that, in general, tissue turnover and thus tooth movement will be slower in the adult patient, particularly in the early stages of treatment.

Individual variations

There is considerable individual variation in the response to orthodontic forces. This is at least in part dependent on the density of the alveolar bone. In some individuals the alveolar bone is cancellous with large marrow spaces, whereas in others it is dense lamellated bone with few marrow spaces. Tooth movement will be much slower in the latter.

Harmful effects of orthodontic tooth movement

Pulp death
This is not common but can result from the application of heavy forces, particularly if the apex of the tooth is closed. It is always wise to proceed cautiously where there is either evidence and/or a history of trauma to the tooth which it is planned to move. In such a situation the blood supply to the pulp may already have been prejudiced.

Root resorption
Minor areas of resorption of cementum on the lateral aspects of the root may be seen during orthodontic tooth movement. These are not important and are usually repaired by cementum. Much more serious is the apical resorption sometimes seen, particularly when teeth have been moved bodily over long distances by fixed appliances. Such root damage may be extensive, but little can be done. In severe cases some may advocate a calcium hydroxide dressing in the root canal to try to arrest the progress of the resorption. If such root resorption is observed during treatment, the tooth movement should be stopped for some months to allow repair by secondary cementum and then, if absolutely necessary, tooth movement may be very carefully recommenced. It is important to recognize that root resorption is not uncommon in patients who have not received orthodontic treatment. For this reason, all teeth to be moved should be radiographed prior to treatment. Where evidence of apical root blunting or alternatively of thin spindly roots is seen on the initial radiographs, the clinician should be aware that these patients are more likely to experience root resorption during orthodontic treatment. If root resorption is observed, one should be very cautious about undertaking treatment and, if necessary, a regular clinical and radiographic review should be maintained during the period that the tooth is loaded.

General conclusions

It is generally thought that only light forces should be used for orthodontic tooth movement. Both vital and non-vital teeth can be moved.

Orthodontic movement is possible only because cementum is more resistant to resorption than bone. Some authors recommend intermittent pressure, some constant pressure. When properly applied, probably little clinical difference exists between the two approaches to treatment.

When excessive force is used, it is very likely that the anchor teeth may move, the amount of force applied to them being ideal to encourage movement of larger rooted teeth. In such a situation the tooth that it is desired to move will often remain stationary due to the excessive force, causing ligament hyalinization and local bone necrosis.

Chapter 14

Removable appliances – construction and use

Removable appliances are orthodontic devices which can be taken out of the mouth by the patient for cleaning. Myofunctional appliances are sometimes referred to as removable appliances in North America and are described in more detail in Chapter 16.

Removable appliances may be active or passive. Active appliances are designed to achieve tooth movement by wire springs or bows, screws, elastics or the acrylic baseplate. Passive appliances are designed to maintain teeth in their present position, e.g. space maintainers or retainers.

Components of removable appliances
* active component
* retention (fixation)
* anchorage
* baseplate.

Some of the components will have a dual function.

Active component

This provides`the force which moves the tooth. This may be derived from wire springs or bows, screws or elastics.

Springs are made from hard stainless steel wire. The simplest spring is the cantilever (Figure 14.1a). The factors affecting the force (F) applied by this spring are given by the expression:

$$F \propto dr^4/l^3$$

i.e. the force is directly proportional to the deflection (d), to the fourth power of the radius (r) and inversely proportional to the cube of the length (l) of the wire. Thus, small variations in the length and particularly in the diameter of the wire will have major effects on the spring characteristics.

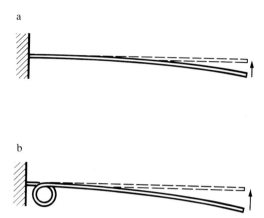

Figure 14.1 a, A simple cantilever. b, The incorporation of a coil increases the deflection of the spring for a given load. Note that the coil should unwind as the tooth moves

A well-designed spring should be most flexible in the direction of activation, but also in other directions. The ratio of these values is termed the stability ratio. A low stability ratio indicates that the spring is liable to be unstable and will be difficult to adjust.

It is usually appropriate to apply a force as light as possible for a given deflection and so the wire should be made as long as possible within the confines of the oral cavity and as thin as is consistent with adequate strength. The effective length of the spring may be increased by incorporating a coil (Figure 14.1b).

For maximum stored energy (i.e. resilience), the coil should unwind as the force is dissipated (Figure 14.1b). This is not always possible with buccal springs. For palatal springs, wire of 0.5 mm diameter may be used, but self-supporting buccal springs should be 0.7 mm in diameter. The spring must be carefully designed so that the tooth will move in the direction intended. The direction of movement is perpendicular to the tangent to the tooth surface at the point of contact of the spring (Figure 14.2). It is very common to find that palatal springs are placed too far back, so that the resultant force is buccally directed. Palatal finger springs are readily distorted and should be protected either by being boxed within a recess of the baseplate or guarded by a length of wire or preferably both (Figure 14.3). The free action of the spring must not be impeded by the box or guards. When adjusting a spring, it is important not to bend it where it emerges from the

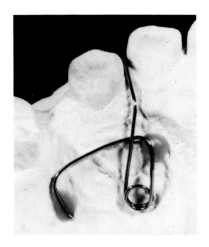

Figure 14.2 A palatal spring with a guard. This spring is positioned so that the tooth will be moved in the line of the arch: the tooth will move perpendicular to the tangent to the surface at the point of contact with the spring

baseplate, otherwise it will fracture in use. Adjustments should be made in the free arm of the spring, taking care that the direction of action is correct. The force applied to a single-rooted tooth should be in the region of 0.3 N. With a typical palatal spring used to retract a canine, an adjustment of about 3 mm (less than one-half of the mesiodistal width of the tooth) will be appropriate. Self-supporting buccal springs (Figure 14.4a) are much more rigid and activation should be correspondingly small (1–2 mm in the case of a typical buccal spring for canine retraction). Their stability ratio is poor. Supported buccal retractors (Figure 14.4b) have a better stability ratio and are more satisfactory in use.

Labial bows (Figure 14.5) are mechanically more complex than springs and their flexibility in the horizontal plane depends to a great extent on the height of any vertical loops incorporated in them. Most unsupported bows are made from 0.7 mm diameter wire but have a poor stability ratio. Supported bows, such as the Roberts retractor (Figure 14.6), are made from 0.5 mm diameter wire. This bow made from thinner wire is very much more flexible, while the stability ratio is favourable.

Screws may be designed to act directly on the teeth through the baseplate (Figure 14.7). A screw applies a large intermittent force to the teeth which is not considered to be the ideal. In most cases screws should be activated, by the patient, one-quarter turn each week. This opens the screw by about 0.2 mm. Thus the tooth movement is small and the periodontal ligament is not crushed.

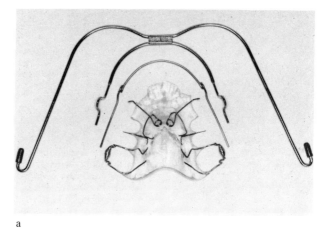

a

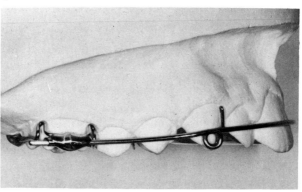

b

Figure 14.3 A simple appliance to retract upper canines with palatal springs. It is usually wise to have tubes attached to the clasps on the molars so that, if required, a facebow (the outer bow) can be fitted to them and anchorage can be reinforced by extra-oral traction worn in the evening and at nights. If a facebow was to be fitted for regular use to the appliance shown, then an anterior clasp on the incisors and a locking catch (see Figure 15.6) would normally be included

As the optimal rate of tooth movement is about 1 mm a month, weekly activation of the screw is usually appropriate. They may also be used to contract dental arches by constructing the appliance with the screw already opened. Screws have the disadvantages that, compared with springs, they are bulky and expensive.

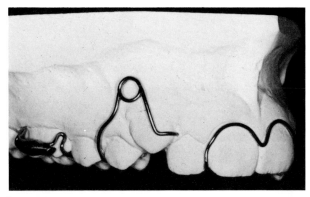

a

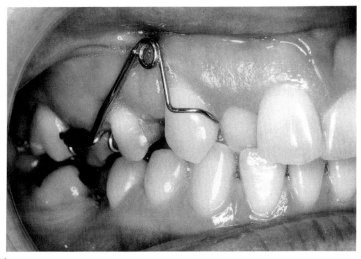

b

Figure 14.4 a, Retraction of a buccally placed canine with a buccally placed spring in 0.7 mm wire. Tubes on the molar clasps provide for the use of extra-oral traction with a facebow if anchorage reinforcement is required. Self-supporting springs like this have a poor stability ratio which makes adjustment difficult. b, Retraction of a buccally placed canine using a supported spring. The wire is 0.5 mm, and distal to the coil is sheathed in 0.5 mm internal diameter tubing. The spring is attached to the appliance by soldering on to the Adams clasp on the first molar. This will allow the canine to be moved distally into contact with the premolar without the thick wire of the sleeving taking up space necessary for correction of the malocclusion

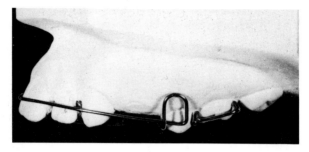

Figure 14.5 Where a small overjet is to be reduced following canine retraction, it may be possible to do this with a labial bow incorporated in the same appliance. This will also prevent any buccal movement of the canines which can be produced by the palatal spring. The stability ratio of this bow is poor

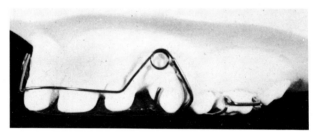

Figure 14.6 A Roberts retractor

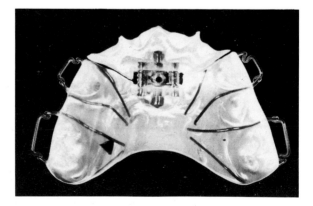

Figure 14.7 A screw plate to procline four upper incisors

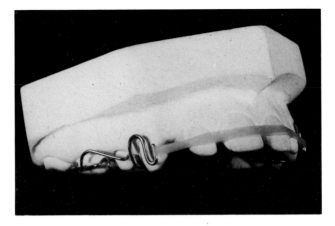

Figure 14.8 The retraction of upper incisors with a latex elastic.
Note: This is not recommended because the elastic tends to slip up
the tooth surface and damage the gingivae

Elastics are usually used as an aesthetic alternative to a wire bow
for reduction of an overjet (Figure 14.8). They are not commonly
used as the active component because they can slide up the labial
surface of the teeth and damage the gingiva. Placement of elastics
directly to teeth (to close a midline diastema, for instance) should
not be carried out as this can lead to severe periodontal damage
and possible loss of the teeth.

Retention or fixation

Retention is the means by which the appliance resists displacement. The term retention is also used to describe the period
following active tooth movement during which the teeth are held
in their new positions while they stabilize (see Chapter 13).
Consequently some prefer the term fixation to describe the resistance to displacement of the plate.

   Retention (fixation) is usually provided by clasps or bows.
Adequate retention can be obtained from Adams clasps on the
molars (Figure 14.9a) and, provided that the incisors are not being
moved by springs, a Southend clasp on the central incisors (Figure
14.9b). Appliances with inadequate retention will be unable to
deliver the correct force to the tooth, will be uncomfortable for
the patient and will encourage poor wear.

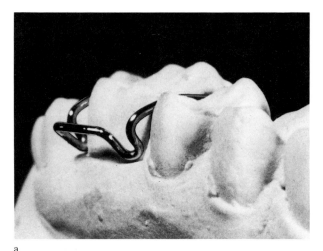

a

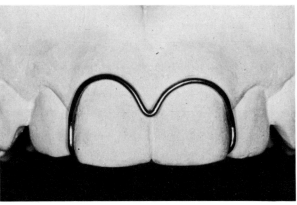

b

Figure 14.9 a, An Adams clasp. Note that the arrowhead engages in undercuts on the mesiobuccal and distobuccal aspects of the molar but does not contact the adjacent teeth. b, A Southend clasp

Remember that teeth to be moved should not have any form of retention or fixation, unless a screw plate is being used, as the clasp will prevent movement. A screw plate is, in effect, two plates joined by a mechanical screw, and both plates will require their own retention. This works well when incisors have to be proclined to correct a Class III incisor relationship. Adjustment of incisor positions in Class II Division 1 malocclusions is achieved by a labial bow which will tend to provide its own retention. Additional retention can be obtained by clasping the canines. This has the advantage of preventing canines moving mesially, but the mesial arm of the clasp may occupy space that is necessary for complete overjet reduction, and modification or removal of the clasp may be necessary in the later stages of treatment.

Anchorage

This is the resistance to the reactive forces generated by the active components of the appliance. Anchorage may be preserved by:

- placement of clasps or bows on teeth which are not being moved
- contact of the baseplate with other teeth not being moved
- contact of the baseplate with the vertical part of the palate in the area of the rugae (for distal movement of teeth)
- use of light forces to move teeth
- movement of a single tooth per quadrant
- intermaxillary elastics (see below)
- extra-oral traction – headgear (see below).

The resistance to tooth movement is related to:

- The surface area of the roots.
- The type of tooth movement permitted: teeth can be tipped more readily than they can be moved bodily. By designing the appliance so that the anchor teeth cannot tip, the anchorage is increased. However, although this is a common practice with fixed appliances, it is not easy with removable appliances.
- Other factors such as the intercuspation of the teeth may contribute to the anchorage.

For descriptive purposes, certain terms are used to classify the various forms of anchorage:

Intramaxillary, where the teeth within the same arch are used as anchorage. This anchorage may be:
Simple, where teeth of greater resistance are used as anchorage for movement of a tooth or teeth of lesser resistance, e.g. pushing an incisor 'over the bite'.
Reciprocal, where two teeth of equal resistance or two equal groups of teeth are used to move each other reciprocally to an equal extent in opposite directions, e.g. transverse arch expansion.

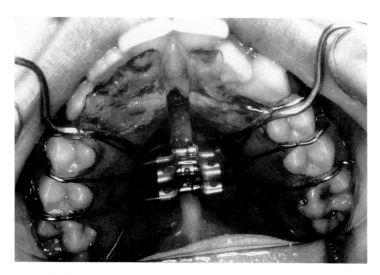

Figure 14.10 An *en masse* appliance for distal movement of the upper buccal segments. Note the midline screw to expand the buccal teeth as they move distally, and Adams clasps on the first molars and premolars to assist retention (fixation)

Intermaxillary, where the opposing arch is used for anchorage. This anchorage may also be simple or reciprocal. Intermaxillary anchorage is most commonly used with fixed appliances where elastics are stretched from the front of one arch to the back of the other (the direction of pull depending on the malocclusion to be treated). However, this is rarely used with removable appliances because the elastics tend to displace the appliances and retention can be a problem.

Extra-oral, where a headcap or neck strap is used to provide or reinforce anchorage (see Figure 15.6). Extra-oral anchorage is a very useful adjunct to removable appliance therapy but appliances must be well made with good retention. The headcap has the advantage over a neck strap in that traction can be directed in a slightly upward direction so that is does not tend to displace the appliance.

When extra-oral anchorage is used as reinforcement to intra-maxillary anchorage, a removable facebow or J hooks are used to transmit the forces to the appliance. The headgear should be worn at night and the force applied should be about twice that provided by the active component of the appliance.

Where anchorage is entirely extra-oral and the force is applied by extra-oral elastics, as in the *en masse* appliance for retraction of upper buccal segments (Figure 14.10), the appliance need be worn only with the headgear. For an acceptable rate of progress, the headgear and appliance must be worn for more than 12 hours out of every 24. Many large-rooted teeth are being moved and so quite heavy forces are appropriate – up to 500 g (about 5 N) in all.

Safety: It should be recognized that it is possible for J hooks or removable facebows to become disengaged, either during play or at night. A few cases have been reported where serious soft-tissue laceration or even damage to an eye has resulted. Various types of safety headgear or safety straps are available to minimize the risk of this happening, and these should be used routinely with J hooks or detachable facebows. Details of these are available from orthodontic suppliers and examples are shown in Chapter 15. To avoid problems of headgear detachment, it is good practice to either design the headgear as an integral part of the appliance or employ an extra-oral bow that locks (see Chapter 15).

Baseplate

This is usually made of cold-cure acrylic which should only be as thick as is consistent with the strength required. A heat-cure acrylic baseplate may be necessary for adults. The baseplate performs the following functions:

- supports the wire or screw components
- contributes to anchorage by contacting teeth not to be moved and the palate
- prevents unwanted drift of teeth
- transmits forces from the active components to the anchorage
- protects palatal springs
- may be extended to form anterior or posterior bite planes.

Anterior bite planes
These are used in order to reduce a deep overbite. They are also useful for relieving occlusal interference with tooth movement in cases where deepening of the overbite (which may occur if posterior planes are used) is to be avoided. Overbite reduction with an anterior bite plane depends largely on occlusal growth of the

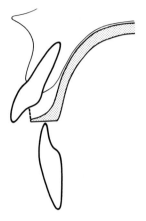

Figure 14.11 Trimming an anterior bite plane to allow incisor retraction. So that the lower incisors will still occlude with it, the bite plane should not be trimmed back too far. Then it is undermined to clear well away from the palatal surface of the upper incisors

posterior teeth which are held out of occlusion, and some minor intrusion of the lower incisors. Anterior bite planes are usually successful in children who have an increased curve of Spee in the lower arch and who have growth remaining.

In Class II cases, overbite reduction should be commenced at the canine retraction stage. The bite plane should exceed the freeway space by 2–3 mm. The bite plane is also useful in removing occlusal interference to canine retraction. When the incisors are retracted, a somewhat thicker plane should be constructed or a low plane may be thickened by additions of cold-cure acrylic. In trimming the bite plane to allow upper incisor retraction (Figure 14.11), it is important to clear it well away from these teeth yet to maintain contact with the lower incisors and provide space for the palatal mucosa to move back. This is because the soft tissues remodel at a much slower rate than the hard tissues. It is useful when designing an appliance to record the size of overjet so that the technician can extend the bite plane by an appropriate amount

Posterior bite planes
These are used to clear occlusal interferences to tooth movement (particularly where there is a mandibular displacement) in appliances for correction of unilateral crossbite (Figure 14.12a) and instanding upper incisors (Figure 14.12b). For comfort, the occlusal coverage of the posterior teeth should be only just thick enough to clear the occlusion.

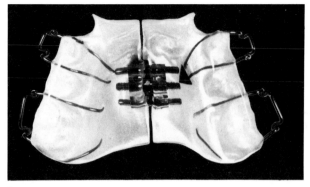

a

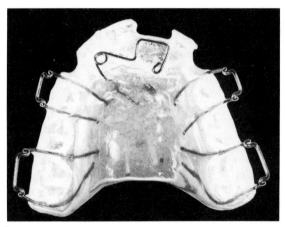

b

Figure 14.12 a, An appliance to expand the upper arch.
Acrylic covering the occlusal surfaces of the premolars and
molars will relieve any cuspal interference from the lower
teeth which may hinder tooth movement. b, An appliance
to procline an instanding incisor with a palatal finger spring.
Note that it is cranked to avoid contact with the other
incisors. Acrylic covering the premolars and molars will
prop the bite open and prevent the incisal overbite from
hindering tooth movement

Construction of removable appliances

Materials used

Stainless steel
In orthodontic work, 18:8 austenitic stainless steel wire is used; in hard form for springs, clasps and arch wires; and in soft form for ligatures and separating wires. It is stainless because the 18% chromium contributes resistance to oxidation by forming a passive surface film and the 8% nickel resists other forms of corrosion. The carbon content is kept as low as practicable (less than 0.5%) as, on heating, chromium carbide tends to be deposited at grain boundaries, reducing corrosion resistance.

Advantages. Cheap, strong, resilient, not affected by the oral fluids, and fairly easy to manipulate.

Disadvantages. Must be worked in hard state, but excessive working causes fatigue and fracture.

Soldering is difficult and requires special flux and even then union is poor. Special fluoride-containing fluxes are necessary to remove the passive surface film of chromium oxide. A low-fusing silver solder is most suitable.

The essential points to be observed are that the wires should be thoroughly cleaned, in close contact and liberally coated with flux. The area of the joint must be adequately heated using a gentle blue flame. The operation should be completed as rapidly as possible to minimize overheating and annealing the adjacent wire.

Welding. In orthodontic spot welding, the pieces to be welded are held together under pressure and a current is passed. The resistance at the junction of the parts results in a rise in temperature and fusion occurs due to localized melting at the point of juncture. The grain structure of the wire should not be seriously affected. A high-density low-voltage current is used (100 A, 5 V) and the time of the weld is made very brief (1/100 sec) to avoid overheating of the wire adjacent to the weld.

Acrylic resin
This is used for the baseplate. Cold-cure acrylic usually has sufficient strength for most removable appliances. This is quicker and more convenient to use than heat-cure acrylic. The latter may be necessary for adults or children with a strong bite. Various coloured acrylics are available which can enhance acceptance of the appliance by the patient.

Construction

Construction of removable appliances will be carried out in the orthodontic laboratory to the prescription of the clinician. It is important that the instructions are clear and unambiguous and that the clinician has a clear idea of what he wants the appliance to achieve. The design should be simple and should not carry too many active components. In addition to a written prescription, a drawing may also be helpful for the technician.

Adams clasps are constructed from 0.7 mm diameter hard stainless steel wire (HSSW) for all except deciduous teeth where 0.5 mm diameter HSSW may be used instead.

Southend clasps are constructed from heat-treated 0.7 mm diameter blue Elgiloy® wire.

Palatally approaching springs which are protected by the baseplate are usually constructed from 0.5 mm diameter HSSW, or 0.7 mm diameter HSSW for molars.

Buccally approaching springs may be self-supporting, in which case they are constructed from 0.7 mm HSSW. Supported buccally approaching springs are constructed from 0.5 mm HSSW which is sheathed up to the coil in 0.5 mm internal diameter stainless steel tubing.

An example of a laboratory prescription card for an appliance to be used in the first stage of the correction of a Class II Division 1 malocclusion, with no anticipated anchorage problems and with the left canine buccally placed and the right canine in arch line, is shown in Figure 14.13.

For details of construction of the various components see Adams and Kerr (1990).

If anchorage reinforcement is required, stainless steel tubes of 1.15 mm internal diameter may be soldered directly to the arm of the Adams clasp, or, to prevent the facebow from acting directly on the clasp and hence reducing its potential retention (fixation), an additional wire may be processed into the baseplate adjacent to the clasp which will carry the tube (Ferguson, 1983). The inner bow of the facebow should match the diameter of the tube, i.e. 1.15 mm diameter wire. The outer bow should be heavier and constructed of 1.5 mm diameter wire.

Indications for removable appliances

The key to all successful orthodontic treatment is a correct diagnosis and treatment plan. When used under the correct

Technician:	**B.H.R.**	Orthodontic Dept Cardiff Dental Hospital	Patients Name:
Date for finish:	17.1.94		Dai Jones 31 Rhondda Street Ynysybwl

Clinician	Staff	✓
	Student	

Study model No.
1 2 3 4

Appliance's function: **URA to retract**   3 | 3   **please**

Instructions:

1   **Adams clasps**   6 | 6   (0.7mm s.s.)
2   **Southend clasp**   1 | 1   (0.7mm Elgiloy)
3   **Palatal cantilever finger spring to retract**   3 | (0.5mm)
4   **Supported buccal canine retractor** | 3   (0.5mm + sleeved)
5   **Anterior bite plane (overjet : 6.0mm)**

Laboratory Card	Date of impression 5.1.94	Patients next App. 19.1.94	Surgeons Sig. **R.G.O.**

Figure 14.13 A laboratory card for an appliance to retract maxillary canines. The right canine is in arch line, but the left canine is buccally placed and therefore needs a buccally approaching spring to correct its position. Note that the patient has a Class II Division 1 malocclusion, and an anterior biting platform has been incorporated into the design to reduce an increased overbite. A second appliance will be necessary to reduce the overjet

circumstances and in competent hands, treatment using removable appliances can provide a simple and economic solution to occlusal problems. Removable appliances are capable of:

- simple tipping movements
- overbite reduction
- elimination of occlusal interferences
- space maintenance/retention
- minor derotations of incisor teeth
- simple extrusion and rotation in conjunction with a fixed attachment.

Simple tipping movements
Teeth tip about a point between one-third and halfway up the root from its apex (see Chapter 13), which means the root apex will move in the opposite direction to the crown. Removable appliances are particularly good at correcting incisor crossbites, provided that the tooth or teeth in crossbite are not already proclined, and there is adequate overbite. A typical appliance design to correct an incisor crossbite would be:

Adams clasps on first permanent molars (0.7 mm HSSW).
Southend clasp (0.7 mm heat-treated blue Elgiloy®) on incisors not being moved, or Adams clasps on deciduous canines (0.5 mm HSSW).
Palatal spring to procline incisors (e.g. either Z spring, T spring, flapper spring, or recurved finger spring, made in 0.5 mm HSSW), boxed by the acrylic.
Posterior bite plane.

It should be remembered that proclination of an incisor will effectively reduce the overbite, and a positive overbite at the end of treatment is essential for stability.

A typical example of an appliance to tip canines or premolars distally is shown in Figure 14.4b.

If a canine is to be tipped distally its initial position must be with excessive mesial tip so that, in its final position, it is ideally still with a mild mesial tip, although an upright position is acceptable. The canine should not finish with its crown distal to the root, as the tooth will suffer unphysiological stresses on the periodontal ligament during function.

Remember also that if distal movement of the mandibular canine is anticipated, then the maxillary canine will have to be moved further distally to achieve or maintain a Class I relationship.

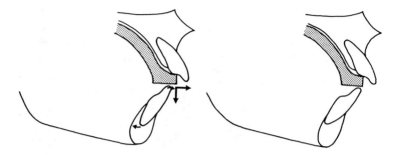

Figure 14.14 The unwanted effects of an anterior biting platform on a removable appliance used in a bimaxillary proclination case. The effect of the biting platform on the lower incisor is to produce a small amount of intrusion, and some further proclination of the tooth. This will be self-limiting when the root meets the lingual cortical plate of bone. The overall effect is an unexpected reduction in overjet caused by lower incisor proclination, which is unstable and liable to relapse when the appliance is withdrawn

Overbite reduction

Incorporation of an anterior bite plane will provide good vertical control in most cases. Anterior biting platforms should not be used to reduce overbite in bimaxillary proclination cases, as their effect will be to procline the mandibular incisors further. Contact of the root apices with the lingual cortical plate of bone in the symphysial area will prevent further bite opening (Figure 14.14; see also Chapter 10).

Elimination of occlusal interferences

Anterior or posterior bite planes will efficiently eliminate occlusal interferences which may hinder crossbite correction. Lower removable appliances with bite planes may also be used to assist a maxillary fixed appliance which is attempting crossbite correction.

Space maintenance/retention

Keeping space in the dental arch for unerupted teeth can be achieved by a variety of means. The advantage of a removable appliance for this purpose is that it can incorporate an anterior bite plane to control the overbite. A further advantage is that it is easy to attach a prosthetic tooth to the baseplate that will not only act as a space maintainer in cases such as congenital absence of a maxillary lateral incisor where space closure is contraindicated, but also enhance aesthetics. A passive removable appliance is frequently used as a retainer following active tooth movement.

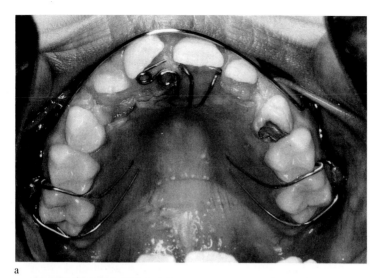

a

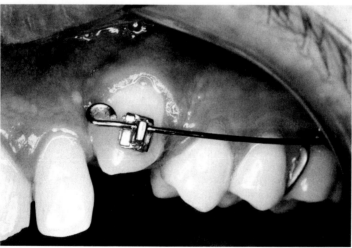

b

Figure 14.15 a, A force couple acting on a rotated central incisor. The palatal Z spring is active on the distopalatal corner and the labial bow is active on the mesiolabial corner of the crown of the tooth. b, Extrusion of a maxillary canine using a combination of a fixed and removable appliance in an adult. A Begg bracket has been directly bonded on to the labial surface of the crown, and a free-ended wire spur in 0.6 mm hard stainless steel wire has been soldered on to the Adams clasp on the first molar. The spur is adjusted to lie just below the level of the incisal edge of the lateral incisor, and is lifted up and placed in the vertical slot of the Begg bracket. This tooth was successfully moved in 3 months

Minor derotations of incisor teeth
A force couple, i.e. two wires acting in opposite directions on diametrically opposed corners of the incisor tooth, will cause derotation (Figure 14.15a). This is only possible if the rotated tooth is upright. Tipped and rotated teeth do not respond well to removable appliance mechanics. Remember that a rotated incisor occupies less space in the arch, and space will be required for derotation.

Simple extrusion and derotation of teeth in conjunction with a fixed attachment
The wide palatal coverage of a removable appliance provides excellent resistance to the reactive forces generated by extrusive mechanics. This can be particularly helpful when straightforward vertical movement of a tooth is necessary. An example of this might be a maxillary canine, or an incisor whose crown has fractured in such a way as to leave the fracture line subgingival. A free-ended spring, with a coil for additional flexibility constructed in 0.5 mm HSSW, hooks over a suitable attachment on the tooth (Figure 14.15b; see also Chapter 15).

Fitting removable appliances

There are several steps involved in fitting an appliance:

1. Before the patient arrives
    (a) Check that you have the correct appliance for the patient.
    (b) Check that the appliance matches the laboratory prescription.
    (c) Check the fit surface of the appliance has no sharp projections (it is often easier to detect these without gloves).
    (d) Check that the appliance fits the model and that the time since the date of the impression is not unacceptably long.
    (e) Check the positioning of the components.
    (f) Check that there is free movement of the active components.
    (g) Check that the headgear bow is a rigid and tight fit to the tubes in the appliance. If there is a locking mechanism (the preferred option), check that it works.
2. With the patient
    (a) Check the fit of the appliance.
    (b) Check and adjust the extension of the baseplate, e.g. trim acrylic from the path of teeth to be moved.

(c) Adjust the active components.
(d) Adjust the retentive components.
(e) Add and adjust headgear if necessary.
(f) Take tooth position measurements, e.g. for retraction of canines measure distance between two reproducible points such as the cusp tip of the canine and the mid-buccal groove of the first molar. Impaling the patient's file with the points of the dividers obviates the need to record the distance in millimetres. Record which landmarks have been chosen. This can be repeated at subsequent visits and comparison made to check progress. Measure overjet (with appliance out of the mouth) and record in the patient's file.
(g) Ask patient if appliance feels comfortable. N.B. If this is the patient's first appliance it will feel strange and a real 'mouthful', but it should not be uncomfortable.
(h) Demonstrate insertion and removal of the appliance with the components in their correct positions to both the patient and parent (if appropriate).
(i) Check that patient can achieve (h) unaided.
(j Give instructions on hours of wear (almost always full-time wear) and cleaning (toothbrush and toothpaste at least once a day). Issue wear chart if necessary. Back up verbal instructions with a written sheet.
(k) Warn patient of initial difficulties in acclimatizing to the appliance, e.g. eating and speaking, and reassure that after 48 hours or so these difficulties will ameliorate. Ask if there are any questions about appliance.
(l) Give subsequent appointment; this will usually be in 4 weeks' time.
3. At the subsequent visit
(a) Ask patient and/or parent about any difficulties with appliance.
(b) Ask patient about wear of appliance. Often the wear of the appliance is dictated by difficulties experienced. If a headgear is fitted, check fit and make sure it does not become detached at night.
(c) Adjust appliance to overcome reported difficulties if necessary.
(d) Repeat measurements to check tooth movement. Between 1 and 2 mm per month movement is satisfactory progress. Untoward overjet increase when moving buccal teeth distally indicates loss of anchorage. See above for methods of preserving anchorage.

(e) Check condition of mouth. Look for marginal gingivitis especially on the palatal aspects adjacent to the baseplate, trauma from the baseplate, retentive or active components and candidal infection beneath the baseplate. Give appropriate advice, prescription or adjustment of appliance.

(f) Reactivate components or, if the tooth movements the appliance was designed to achieve have occurred, then stop treatment or take an impression for the next appliance. Remember at this stage to keep the current appliance passive so that the new appliance will fit.

(g) Tell patient (and parent) of progress, or lack of progress.

(h) Give subsequent appointment.

Appliance not being worn

There are several signs which can indicate that the appliance is not being worn:

1. There is little or no tooth movement.
2. The appliance still looks new. The baseplate retains its high polish, and does not become cloudy due to absorption of oral fluids.
3. The patient's speech is affected when the appliance is in the mouth.
4. The patient has difficulty removing and, more importantly, inserting the appliance.
5. The springs are still active.
6. The appliance may not fit well as there may have been tooth movement when the appliance was out of the mouth.
7. There will be no imprint of the arrowhead of the Adams clasp on the gingivae.
8. There will be no outline of the shape of the baseplate on the palate.
9. The patient may admit to not wearing the appliance. Possible reasons for this include
    (a) instructions misunderstood
    (b) pain or discomfort
    (c) appliance broken/lost
    (d) appearance
    (e) dislike/intolerance of appliance.

The clinician should identify the cause for lack of wear and attend to the problem. It is important that both patient and parent realize the importance of compliance with appliance wear.

Unsuccessful appliance therapy

This may be due to poor compliance (see above), iatrogenic factors and intrinsic patient factors.

Iatrogenic factors
1. Incorrect choice of treatment mechanics, i.e. attempting to correct a malocclusion using the wrong type of appliance.
2. Incorrect choice of extractions. This usually means extraction of second premolars rather than first premolars and having insufficient space to achieve full alignment. The reverse can also be true, with too much space being left at the end of treatment.
3. Poor anchorage control.
4. Incorrect appliance design. Although a removable appliance might be suitable for correction of the malocclusion, incorrect design will hinder progress.
5. Poor fit of appliance, leading to patient discomfort. May be due to overlong period between taking impression and fitting appliance. This problem of fit may be compounded if extractions have been performed in the interim. Normally a removable appliance should be fitted within 1 month of taking the impression, and preferably sooner if extractions have been carried out.
6. Baseplate trimmed incorrectly. Failure to clear acrylic from the path of the advancing tooth, or to appreciate the bunching-up of soft tissues in front of the tooth can prevent tooth movement.
7. Too many active components. The appliance should be designed to move only a small number of teeth. It is preferable to use two or more appliances to achieve correction than to try incorporating all the components into one appliance.
8. Active components incorrectly adjusted. Too much activation of springs, etc., is likely to cause loss of anchorage because the reaction to the heavy force on the tooth to be moved will be a light (optimal) force on the anchor teeth, encouraging their movement (see Chapter 13).
9. Retentive (fixation) components ineffective. This will allow displacement of the appliance with a reduction in efficiency of the spring and will be uncomfortable for the patient.
10. Trauma. Incorrectly placed or adjusted springs can cause trauma, which, in turn, will not encourage appliance wear.
11. Wrong instructions given to the patient regarding appliance wear.

12. Unstable end-point of treatment. If the teeth have been moved into an unstable position there will, without permanent retention, always be relapse.

Intrinsic patient factors
In spite of a correctly designed, constructed, adjusted and worn appliance, teeth may still fail to move. This may be because the tooth is ankylosed, e.g. a previously traumatized incisor that has healed by ankylosis. There is nothing that can be done to move this tooth. There may be an area of sclerotic bone in the path of the tooth. This may be the result of a difficult extraction.

There may be anatomical limitations. Teeth can only be moved where there is bone. Severe skeletal discrepancies will require a combination of surgery and orthodontics to overcome these problems (see Chapter 19). At a local level, loss of alveolar bone will lead to a narrowing of the channel of cancellous bone through which the tooth can move easily (see Figure 6.5).

Chapter 15

Fixed appliances

Fixed appliances are powerful and complex mechanisms and their unskilled use may lead to extensive and rapid unwanted tooth movements. The dental practitioner without special training should not attempt to use fixed appliances. However, he may need to refer patients requiring fixed appliance treatment to an orthodontic specialist. Thus he should have some knowledge of their scope and action.

Definition. A fixed appliance is an orthodontic device where attachments are fixed to the teeth and forces applied by arch wires or auxiliaries through these attachments. This allows precise three-dimensional control over the nature and direction of the forces applied.

Components of fixed appliances

Attachments

The attachments (brackets, tubes, etc.) are peculiar to each fixed appliance technique. Their function is to allow a controlled force (or couple of forces) to be applied to the tooth (Figure 15.1). The attachments may be directly fixed to the teeth by means of

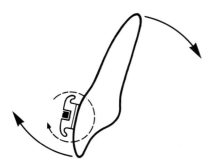

Figure 15.1 A mechanical couple can be applied to a tooth with a fixed appliance. This means that precise control over root movement is possible

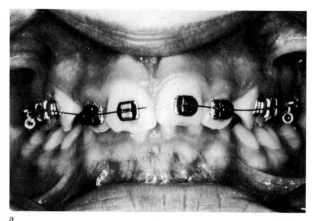

a

b

Figure 15.2 An Edgewise appliance with directly bonded
attachments. a, A thin diameter round wire is used to obtain
initial alignment of the teeth and, b, precise control of tooth
positions is achieved by the use of rectangular archwires. The
loops in this latter wire are active components designed to
retract the incisors and reduce the overjet

etch-retained composite resin (Figure 15.2) or some similar
system. Alternatively, the attachment may be welded to stainless
steel bands which are then in turn cemented to the teeth. Bands
may be purchased in a variety of stock sizes or may be individually constructed from stainless steel tape. Directly bonded attachments are generally less conspicuous than bands, but during

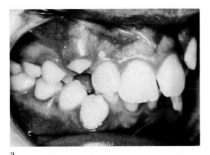

a

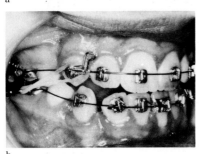

b

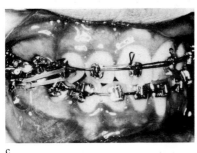

c

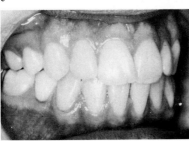

d

Figure 15.3 A Begg appliance.
The brackets have vertical slots
which accommodate soft metal
pins to hold the archwire in place.
a, Prior to treatment. b, After
initial alignment of the teeth with
looped arches, plain arches are
used in conjunction with
intermaxillary elastics to close
space and attain an edge-to-edge
incisor relationship. c, In a later
stage of treatment, apical
movements of the teeth are made
to correct their inclinations.
These are achieved by auxiliary
attachments and springs. d,
Finished result (Records of this
case by courtesy of Mr R. Edler)

bonding, the tooth must be kept absolutely dry. They are used on anterior teeth, whereas molars, particularly if extra-oral traction is to be applied, are usually banded.

Archwires

Depending on the technique, round or rectangular archwires may be used and are fixed to the brackets by soft wire ligatures, elastomeric rings or pins. The archwire may be active (the archwire is deflected on tying in to the attachments so that forces are applied to the teeth), or passive (the archwire is not deflected but forces are applied by auxiliary springs or elastics). Active archwires often have loops bent into them (Figure 15.3b) to increase their flexibility at sites of irregularity or where spaces have to be opened or closed.

Auxiliaries

Forces may be applied to the teeth by auxiliary springs or elastics. As an example latex elastics are used for transmitting forces between the arches (intermaxillary traction) as well as within the one arch (intramaxillary traction).

Advantages and disadvantages of fixed compared with removable appliances

Fixed
- Precise control over force distribution to individual teeth means that rotation and controlled root movement are possible.
- Multiple tooth movements can be performed simultaneously.
- Complex to make and use, so special training is needed.
- Chairside time is comparatively long.
- Components are usually more costly (this is now less of a problem).
- Oral hygiene is made more difficult.

Removable
- Single-point application of forces means that only tipping movements are readily produced.
- Usually only a few teeth should be moved at any one time. The appliance should be kept as simple as possible.

- Treatment should be kept comparatively simple and should be within the scope of the dental practitioner.
- Only suitable for carefully selected cases.
- Chairside time is usually short, but laboratory time is generally greater than for fixed appliances.
- Components are usually inexpensive and easy to obtain.
- Since the appliance is removable, the problems of oral hygiene should not be any more increased than normal.

Limitations of fixed appliances

It should be recognized that many of the limitations of removable appliance treatment apply equally to fixed appliances.

1. Patient co-operation is required, even though the appliance is fixed. The unco-operative patient will not maintain an adequate standard of oral hygiene, will not wear intra-oral elastics or headgear as directed and may intentionally or carelessly damage his appliances. Thus, fixed appliance treatment is not appropriate for the unco-operative child who will not wear removable appliances. Indeed, in general, a similarly high level of co-operation is required whatever type of orthodontic appliance is selected.
2. The rate of tooth movement is limited by the biological response of the supporting tissues. This is the same, regardless of the type of appliance used.
3. Treatment effects are limited to the teeth and alveolar structures. While it is possible by controlled tooth movement with fixed appliances to obtain good occlusion even where the skeletal relationship is unfavourable, the improvement in the patient's facial appearance may not match the improvement in occlusion. Where the skeletal pattern is very adverse, it is not possible to obtain a good occlusion, even with fixed appliances. In such situations, surgery would be required to correct both the skeletal discrepancy and improve the facial profile.
4. Stability of treatment with fixed appliances depends on exactly the same factors as with removable appliances: the position of balance depends on the harmonious interaction between skeletal relationship, soft-tissue pattern and interdental forces. Having stated this, multiple tooth movement is possible with a fixed appliance and therefore careful consideration should be given to the retention phase. In particular, teeth with large rotations are prone to relapse: such corrections should be made early and retained for longer.

Fixed appliance techniques

Multiband techniques

A variety of techniques is available in which attachments are fitted to most or all of the teeth. Archwires are designed so that controlled tooth movement in any plane of space is possible. The most widely known fixed appliance systems are based on the Edgewise and the Begg techniques.

Edgewise technique

This technique is based on a method for moving teeth first described by Edward Angle, the father of modern orthodontics (1928). Attachments with rectangular slots are used (Figure 15.2). Light, small-diameter, round wires may be fitted for initial alignment, but for controlled tooth movement in all planes of space rectangular archwires, which more closely fit the corresponding slot in the bracket, are used.

Begg technique

In contrast with the Edgewise technique, the attachments have simple vertical slots which allow free tipping of the teeth (Figure 15.3). Round archwires are used and controlled root movement in any direction is obtained by the use of auxiliary springs (Begg and Kesling, 1977).

Treatment stages
Whichever technique is selected, treatment may be divided into four main phases:

1. *Alignment phase.* During this initial phase crowding and rotations are rapidly dealt with to allow the placement of more rigid working archwires. Very flexible wires with large working ranges are used during this early part of treatment. In the past, multiple loops might have been bent into a steel wire to allow the distraction of the archwire into the brackets on malpositioned teeth; it is more common in current practice to use thin, twisted (braided/multiflex) steel or preformed superelastic nickel–titanium alloy wires, both of which are very efficient at gaining initial tooth alignment with reduced chairside time.
2. *Working phase.* During this middle period of treatment, horizontal and vertical dento-alveolar corrections are made. Thus the overbite and overjet are reduced. During this phase

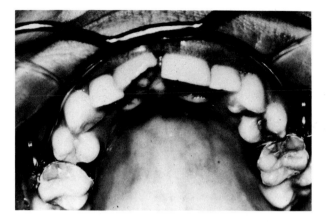

Figure 15.4 Bands cemented to first permanent molars carry
tubes into which the ends of the facebow can be fitted. This,
together with the headgear, is worn at nights or as prescribed.
Some form of safety headgear should always be used (see text)

a more rigid archwire is employed, along which the teeth (via
the brackets) are generally moved. All spaces are eliminated.
3. *Finishing phase.* Larger archwires more closely fitting the
bracket slot are placed. Tooth position is carefully detailed to
achieve the best aesthetic and functional result.
4. *Retention phase.* The fixed appliance is removed and usually
retainers are fitted. These, in contemporary practice, are most
usually upper and lower removable appliances designed to
tightly fit around the incisors and hold any corrected rotations.
The retainers are worn full time for 4–6 months, then at night-
time only for 4–6 months. Since they are removable they can
then gradually be withdrawn a little at a time to test for tooth
stability. There is no absolute rule with regard to a retention
regimen, every case being treated on its merits. On occasion,
fixed retainers may be appropriate. These are most commonly
employed in the region of the lower incisors, where they might
be bonded to the lingual surfaces of the lower permanent
canines.

Fixed–removable appliances

Sometimes it is useful to be able to use fixed attachments in
association with a removable appliance. As an example, where the

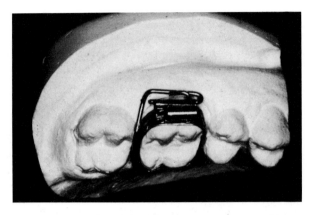

Figure 15.5 A modified molar clasp for an upper removable appliance to be worn in conjunction with the bands on the molars

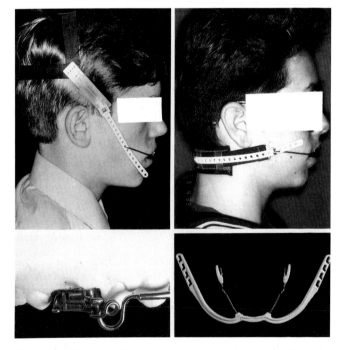

Figure 15.6 Various methods for improving headgear safety. Top left to bottom right: snap-release, anti-recoil strap, locking catch between inner bow and molar buccal tube, plastic covering all wire ends (By courtesy of Mr R. Samuels)

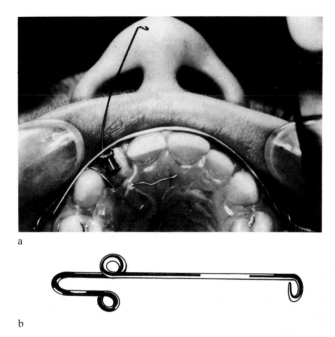

a

b

Figure 15.7 a, A whip on the upper lateral incisor with a directly bonded Edgewise bracket. b, Design of the whip which is made from 0.5 mm wire. It clips over the wings of the bracket and is held in place by a ligature twisted through the loops in the wire. The free end of the whip clips over the labial bow and a rotational couple is applied to the tooth. The patient can take out the removable appliance for cleaning (Compare this with Figure 14.15)

retention of a removable is liable to be poor and it is desirable to use extra-oral traction, bands may be cemented direct to upper molars to carry a facebow (Figure 15.4). This can be used alone to retract the upper molars or to reinforce anchorage in conjunction with a removable appliance. In that case, modified clasps to fit over the tubes on the molar bands are used on the appliance (Figure 15.5). In either situation, it is wise to incorporate safety mechanisms to reduce the risks of recoil and resultant injuries which may affect the face or, in more serious circumstances, the eyes. Such injuries are often due to an incorrect headgear removal procedure, horseplay by the patient or detachment of facebows during sleep. A number of safety mechanisms are available (Figure 15.6); however, they do not reduce the need for careful

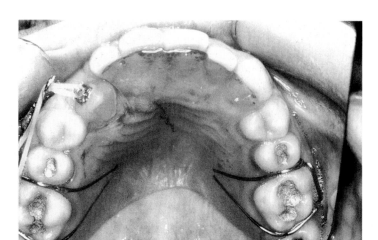

a

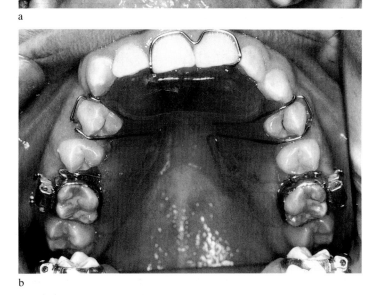

b

Figure 15.8 a, A removable/fixed appliance for moving a canine where the crown is palatal but the root apex is favourably positioned. b, A removable appliance to support distal movement of upper molars with extra-oral traction. Springs should be only lightly activated (Case by courtesy of Mr J. Buckley)

instructions on fitting and any patient experiencing detachment of headgear should return to the clinician as soon as possible. ·

Where one or perhaps two incisors are rotated, a whip and bonded attachment may be effective when used in conjunction with a labial bow from a removable appliance (Figure 15.7), although a local fixed appliance generally gives better control. By similar means a favourably inclined canine may be drawn across the occlusion from a palatal position (Figure 15.8a). In both of these examples, directly bonded attachments are useful, being connected to the tooth to be moved by the conventional acid/etch technique.

An upper removable appliance may also be used in the early stages of a standard fixed appliance treatment, an anterior bite plane assisting bite opening or clearing the occlusion to allow early lower incisor bracket placement. Gently activated springs mesial to molars may assist the distal movement of these teeth by extra-oral traction (Figure 15.8b).

Segmental fixed appliances

These constitute locally applied fixed appliances generally used in isolation in a buccal or labial segment of the dental arch to improve the tooth alignment. They often form part of an adjunctive treatment (see Chapter 20).

Preadjusted fixed appliances

Edgewise

In recent years, preadjusted versions of the Edgewise appliance have become popular. In such systems, instead of having a simple slot cut in the Edgewise bracket and making adjustments to the tooth position by placing bends or twists in the archwire, the tooth correction is built into the bracket slot and/or base. An individual bracket is available for each tooth and carries the average correction for angulation and inclination (torque). Varying the thickness of the bracket base allows the 'in/out' relationship of each tooth to the arch form to be considered. As an example, the average tendency of an upper lateral incisor to be more palatal than the neighbouring central incisor is reflected in a thicker bracket base for the lateral. This detail, which is built into every individual bracket, means that flat archwires, of a set curve

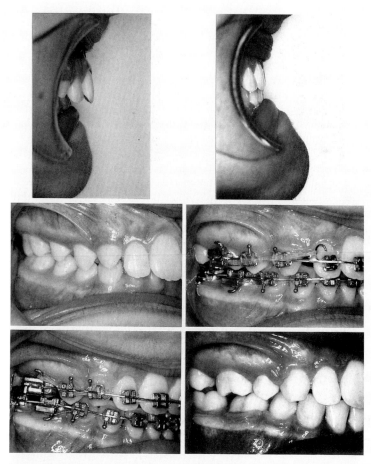

Figure 15.9 A case treated by means of the Roth prescription 'Straight-Wire Appliance', a preadjusted Edgewise appliance employing full arch mechanics. Middle left to lower right shows sequence of mechanics for a moderate Class II Division 1 case. Note the overjet reduction by means of sliding mechanics along the archwire, the force being provided by intramaxillary elastic traction while the anchor molars are held in position by headgear. The upper views show start to finish overjet (Records by courtesy of Mr J. Knox)

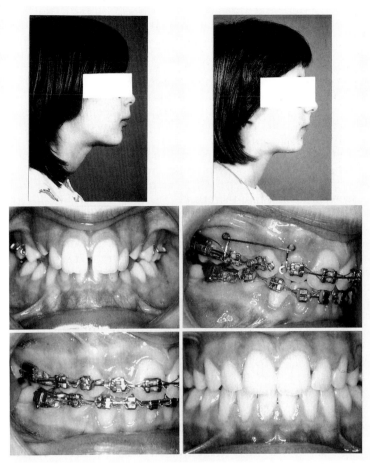

Figure 15.10 A case treated by means of the Bioprogressive technique – a version of preadjusted Edgewise appliance employing sectional mechanics. Middle left to lower right shows the sequence of mechanics. Initially a space maintainer has been fitted both to hold space following extraction and to start bite opening. After the upper canines have erupted they have been retracted using a sectional archwire (see also Figure 20.3). Next the overjet has been reduced using another section termed a 'utility'. Finally, full archwires have been fitted to respond to the prescription in the bracket and facilitate individual tooth positioning. The upper views show the before and after facial profile (Records by courtesy of Ms H. Taylor)

(preformed in the factory), may be fitted with the minimum of adjustment straight from the packet. In particular such systems facilitate the use of superelastic alloy which have a 'shape memory' and improved flexibility. The advantage of such systems lies in the saving in clinical time and the improved consistency of a good finished result. The disadvantages include cost, the increased stock necessary and the need for the clinician to recognize the occasional cases where a set prescription in the bracket or archwire is inappropriate.

It is important in any type of fixed appliance mechanism to correctly position the bracket on the crown of the tooth; this is an especially important factor when the main prescription for tooth movement is built into the bracket.

Popular types of Edgewise preadjusted appliances include the systems described by Andrews (1979) or alternatively Roth. These two systems only differ in the prescription built into the bracket and base. A case treated by the Roth prescription appliance is shown in Figure 15.9. Another approach is to treat the case in the early stages by sectional arches and then, when the main corrections have been achieved, fit full arches in a similar manner to conventional Edgewise to finish. An example of such a system is the Bioprogressive technique, as developed by Ricketts (1976) . Its advantage lies in minimizing the effects of friction while allowing a careful balance of anchorage to be maintained. Its disadvantage lies in the difficulty in controlling tooth movements, especially during the early stages of treatment. Figure 15.10 shows a case treated by this technique. A fuller description of the technique is available elsewhere (Jones et al., 1992).

Begg

A preadjusted version of the Begg appliance is also available, called Tip-Edge. In this system the early stages of treatment follow conventional lines (see Figure 15.3). However, the bracket includes a preadjusted element, similar to the Edgewise bracket, which facilitates the fitting of a rectangular finishing wire at the end of treatment.

Chapter 16

Functional appliances

Functional appliances utilize the forces of the orofacial musculature to move teeth. The fact that they depend on muscle forces
in no way implies a special mode of action: they largely produce
their effects as a result of tooth movement brought about by the
tissue changes described in Chapter 13. The major effect of
functional appliances is on the position of the teeth and alveolar
processes, in other words the correction of the malocclusion is
largely by dento-alveolar camouflage. There is still much debate
about the possibility of orthopaedic change, with some evidence
that in favourable cases mandibular condylar growth may be
modified or redirected.

Many functional appliances have been described but only the
more important examples from each group will be mentioned in
this text. For a more detailed account of their use and construction see Houston *et al.* (1992), Adams and Kerr (1990) or Orton
(1990).

The Oral Screen

This early simple functional appliance is now largely of historical
interest but is still used on occasions. The appliance (Figure 16.1)
consists of a thin shield of acrylic which lies in the buccal sulcus.
It is worn at night. In its passive form it transmits the forces of
the circumoral musculature uniformly to the teeth. The passive
oral screen has been used as a retainer (following upper incisor
retraction in Class II Division 1 cases) and to discourage thumb
sucking. It has also been used in an attempt to reduce night-time
drying of the upper gingivae in patients with local inflammation
associated with lip incompetence.

In its active form it contacts only the upper incisors and stands
away from the other teeth so that the muscular forces are concentrated on the upper incisors. The passive screen may be made
active by adding a thin layer of cold-cure acrylic to the screen

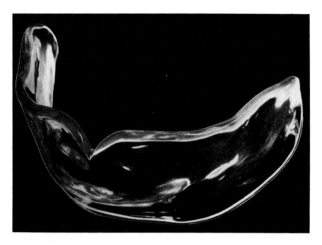

Figure 16.1 An Oral Screen

where it contacts the upper incisors. The active oral screen has been used for overjet reduction in cases where there is sufficient incisor spacing and the overbite is incomplete so that the lower incisors do not interfere with the upper incisor retraction. It is probably fair to say that the same result can be obtained more quickly and with less inconvenience to the patient by a more conventional removable appliance.

In its active form there is a danger of applying an excessive, although admittedly intermittent, force to the upper incisors.

The Andresen appliance

This appliance (Figure 16.2a) was developed from the monobloc of Robin (1902). It consists of upper and lower appliances sealed together with the mandibular arch postured, so that the forces of the muscles of mastication can be transmitted between the arches. This produces an intermaxillary type of force which acts to correct the Class II type of anteroposterior arch discrepancy.

Although a variety of malocclusions may be treated by the expert, the general use of the Andresen appliance is confined to carefully selected Class II Division 1 cases with the following classically described features:

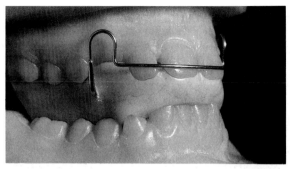

a

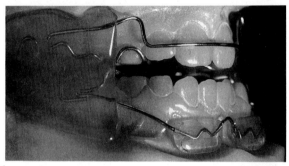

b

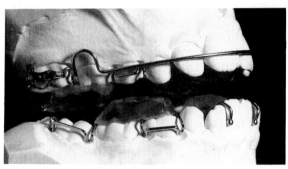

c

Figure 16.2 a, An Andresen appliance. The bite has been postured forwards in this Class II Division 1 case – in this instance it is more open than classically described. b, A Fränkel appliance. The bite has been postured forwards into the appliance to correct the Class II Division 1 malocclusion. c, Clark's Twin Block appliance. In this adaptation of the appliance, headgear tubes are also included. The models have been opened for the purposes of illustration in this Class II Division 1 case

- The arches must be uncrowded and in regular alignment. It is advantageous if the lower incisors are spaced. The upper molars must not be inclined distally.
- The lower arch should not normally be more than one-half cusp width distal to the upper.
- The skeletal pattern should be ideally Class I or mild Class II.
- There must be no habit posture of the mandible.
- Ideally the patient should not have entered their prepubertal growth spurt.

For success, the working bite and laboratory procedures must be carried out carefully. The working bite is taken with the mandible. symmetrically postured forwards to obtain a Class I buccal segment relationship and opened about 2 mm beyond the freeway space. This means that when the appliance is fitted, the mandible is held forwards and the muscles acting on it (in particular the posterior fibres of temporalis) tend to retract it to its normal position. As a result, forces are generated which tend to move the upper teeth distally and the lower teeth mesially. This is an example of intermaxillary traction. In order to facilitate tooth movement and allow overbite reduction, channels are trimmed over the occlusal surfaces of the molars and premolars. These channels are directed backwards in the upper arch and forwards in the lower. As a result, the appliance contacts the upper posterior teeth only on their mesiopalatal aspects and the lowers only on their distolingual aspects. This guides their direction of eruption to encourage correction of the occlusion. It is important that, in the construction of the appliance, the acrylic should be carried over the lower incisor tips. The capping acts as a bite plane to permit overbite reduction and is meant to prevent the lower incisors from tipping forwards. However, a major problem with the Andresen appliance is that the lower incisors may be moved labially out of muscle balance and therefore could relapse when treatment is completed.

The patient is instructed to wear the appliance at night and for as many hours as possible each day. With careful case selection good results may be obtained, but the clinician needs to make a careful assessment of the facial profile before prescribing a functional appliance: where a true maxillary protrusion is present, such cases may more readily be treated by using a more conventional appliance. For example, the mild uncrowded Class II Division I malocclusion may be treated by using extra-oral traction to retract the upper buccal segments, followed by overjet reduction, without any risk of disturbing the balance of the lower arch.

The Harvold appliance

This appliance, which is also known as the Harvold Activator (Harvold and Vargevick, 1971) belongs to a group of essentially tooth-borne appliances which all derive from the original design of Andresen. It differs in that it holds the teeth further apart, thus exhibiting a greater potential for both bite-opening and inter-maxillary traction. It is also trimmed differently in that the appliance's lingual flange is constructed to be well clear of the teeth of the lower buccal segments: this allows the teeth of the lower buccal segments to erupt upwards and forwards to assist both the overbite and the horizontal molar correction.

The very large amount of vertical opening is intended to take advantage of a theoretical muscular and soft-tissue recoil to correct the Class II arch relationship. However, such a degree of opening can also make the appliance uncomfortable to wear.

The Fränkel appliance

This is a variety of functional appliance (Figure 16.2b) which differs from the Andresen appliance in that its action primarily depends on acrylic shields which are designed to hold the lips and cheeks away from the teeth, so disturbing the muscle balance and producing tooth movement. This appliance has been described as being soft-tissue-borne rather than tooth-borne, the latter being the case with most other appliances in the family of functionals. In Class II cases, the appliance is designed to hold the mandible in a forward position. The appliance is described by Fränkel (1980) as a 'function regulator' (FR) and, as its name implies, he believes that it permanently modifies the position and activities of the orofacial muscles and promotes growth at the mandibular condyle. At the present time there is no objective evidence to support these concepts. Treatment with the Fränkel appliance is usually begun in the early mixed dentition. The appliance is worn part time until the patient is accustomed to it, then full time. Although the appropriate design of Fränkel appliance theoretically can be used to treat any arch malrelationship, it is used most commonly in Class II Division 1 malocclusions. Crowding in Class II cases is not a contraindication to its use, since some arch expansion is produced, but clearly the result will not be stable unless the teeth are in a position of muscle balance at the end of treatment.

Clark's Twin Block appliance

This tooth-borne functional appliance has become very popular in recent years for the treatment of moderate to severe Class II Division 1 type malocclusions. It differs from the Andresen in that the upper and lower components of the appliance are not sealed together, being free to move apart when the patient opens the mouth. On closure (Figure 16.2c), angled posterior bite blocks on the upper and lower plates guide the occlusion into a postured position, similar to that obtained with other functionals. The principal advantage of the twin block is that it is better tolerated than most functionals and is therefore worn for longer hours to achieve a more rapid correction of the anteroposterior arch discrepancy. As with other functional appliances, it is usually unwise to attempt a full horizontal occlusal correction in one go. Accordingly, the mandibular arch should not be initially postured forwards by much more than 7 mm, otherwise the appliance may prove uncomfortable and will not be worn. Clark's appliance may be activated quite easily during treatment by adding acrylic to the blocks (Clarke, 1988).

In both the Clark and Fränkel appliance the likely effect on the facial profile of a successful treatment may be rehearsed by asking the patient to posture the mandible forwards to a Class I incisor relationship.

Conclusion

A very large number of functional appliances have been described in the literature, but unfortunately there have been very few scientifically valid studies to investigate how they achieve correction of the malocclusion. However, it would appear that much of the change in dental arch relationship is achieved by a combination of dento-alveolar camouflage and favourable growth of the jaws. For the best chance of success, the appliance must be worn for long hours and the treatment timed to coincide with the individual's growth spurt. Since both of these factors are, to a large extent, outside the control of the clinician, it is wise to review progress carefully. If little change is seen after 6 months it would probably be sensible to consider other possible treatment options.

At their most effective, functional appliances are very valuable in that they provide a possible treatment in the mixed dentition for significant horizontal dental arch discrepancies. Although they may be employed in other types of malocclusion, they appear to be most useful in Class II Division 1 types. Once the overjet is corrected, a fixed appliance can be fitted subsequently to allow the correction of any crowding.

Chapter 17

Radiology in orthodontics

The importance and value of radiographs in diagnosis and treatment planning is well documented. However, a radiograph should never be taken unless it offers a 'benefit' to the patient that 'outweighs the risk' of the radiation exposure. Therefore, as for all medical and dental practitioners, the orthodontic clinician should be able to justify the taking of each radiograph as being to the advantage of the individual patient. Taking a radiograph cannot be justified on medicolegal grounds alone.

This chapter gives a brief account of the main projections used in orthodontics, the main clinical indications for radiography, together with some recommendations to assist the clinician in matching the appropriate view with the information required. Bearing in mind the biological effects and risks of X-rays, the practitioner has ethical and legal obligations to minimize the radiation dose to patients, to himself, to his staff and to the public at large.

The nature and source of X-rays

X-rays are a form of high-energy (short-wavelength) electromagnetic radiation and are part of the electromagnetic spectrum, which also includes low-energy (long-wavelength) radio waves and visible light.

There are two main sources of radiation – natural and artificial. The natural sources (cosmic rays and certain rock emissions) contribute 87% of the background radiation, while the remaining 13% are of artificial origin. The vast majority of this latter group (12%) is generated for medical purposes. The average dose from background radiation is estimated at approximately 2.5 millisieverts (mSv) per year for each inhabitant of the UK.

Radiation quantities

The main X-ray beam is dependent for *intensity* on the quantity and quality of radiation. The *quantity* (number of photons) is

Table 17.1   Terms and units in X-ray dosimetry

Quantity	Old unit	New SI unit	
Absorbed dose	rad	Gray (Gy) (1 Gy = 100 rad)	Amount of energy absorbed per unit mass of tissue (joules/kg)
Dose equivalent	rem	sievert (Sv) (1 Sv = 100 rem)	Takes into account the radio/biological effectiveness (RBE) of different types of radiation (Quality factor= Q: for X-rays, $Q = 1$; for alpha particles, $Q = 20$)
Effective dose equivalent	rem	sievert (Sv)*	Dose equivalent × weighting factor (W) (each tissue has been allocated a numerical value, based on its radiosensitivity)
Collective dose equivalent		man-sievert	Effective dose equivalent × population

*Subunits: millisieverts (mSv = Sv × 10^{-3}; microsieverts μSv = Sv × 10^{-6}).

influenced by the milliamperage (mA) of the X-ray apparatus and the length of the exposure time, whereas the *quality* (energy of photons and penetration power) of X-rays is influenced by kilovoltage (kV).

It is important to understand the various terms and units used in dosimetry in order to appreciate the meaning of *radiation dose*. These are summarized in Table 17.1.

The *absorbed dose* measures the amount of energy imparted by radiation to a unit mass of tissue. It is expressed in a unit of measurement termed the *gray* (Gy). Since equal absorbed doses from various radiations (e.g. X-rays, alpha particles) do not necessarily have equal biological effects, another quantity is needed. This is the dose equivalent which is expressed in a unit of measurement called the *sievert* (Sv). Dose equivalent is equal to the absorbed dose multiplied by a factor that takes account of the way a particular radiation distributes energy in tissue, thus influencing its effectiveness in causing harm. A further consideration in examining the dose with regard to the risk of fatal malignancy or hereditary damage per sievert is that it is not the same for all tissue types. As an example, it is lower for the thyroid than for the testes or ovaries. For this reason, the dose equivalent in each

Table 17.2   Typical effective dose from dental and some medical examinations, the estimated risk of fatal cancer per million examinations and equivalent natural background radiation

X-ray examination	Effective dose (mSv)	Estimated risk per million of a fatal cancer	Equivalent period of natural background radiation
Dental intra-oral (2 bitewings)	0.002*	0.01	8 hours
R. and L. oblique lateral	0.015	0.09	
Dental panoramic tomograph	0.007*	0.04	28 hours
Collimated lateral ceph.	0.015	0.09	2.5 days
Skull	0.1	6.0	17 days
Chest	0.04	0.2	7 days
Barium meal	4.6	265	2.1 years

*The dose for IO and OPT varies by a factor of up to 50 times.
The above values were obtained by using E speed film, rectangular collimation and rare-earth screens.

of the major organs and tissues of the body is subject to a weighting factor related to the individual risk to that organ. The sum of these corrected measurements is termed the *effective dose equivalent* and it is recorded in sieverts.

The word 'dose' is applied loosely to the effective dose equivalent and the subunits millisievert (mSv) and microsievert (μSv) may be used. The average radiation dose from different radiological examinations, together with estimated risk and equivalent period of natural background radiation, are given in Table 17.2.

Risk estimation

The effects of low-dose radiation are demonstrable only as a statistical increase in the frequency of normally increasing disease, for example fatal cancer, among the general population. Risk estimation can be expressed in two ways: the first is the difference between the risk in an irradiated compared to a non-irradiated population, and the second estimation is made on the basis of per million radiographic examinations.

No dose of radiation can be considered as safe, no matter how small. However, the small risks involved in dental radiography should be kept in perspective.

General measures to minimize exposure dose and risks

In addition to the use of well-maintained and monitored X-ray equipment and a high standard of radiographic technique, the operator must never stand in the direct line of the main beam. It is best to stand behind a lead barrier or no closer than 1.5 m (6 ft) to the unit during an exposure and preferably at right angles to the beam. The following general measures should also be followed.

Selection criteria
Prescription of radiographs should be based on the history and clinical findings, and they must only be undertaken when the investigation is likely to affect the management of the patient in terms of diagnosis and treatment. Decisions should be based on the information required. Important factors are:

- the likely abnormality being investigated and its extent
- whether a general or detailed view is necessary
- whether the patient is new to the clinic or has been recalled
- whether special radiological or scanning techniques are indicated.

The frequency with which films are taken will depend on the availability/timing of previous radiographs together with any monitoring regimen that is being pursued. However, it is important that radiography is not seen as a 'routine' procedure that automatically accompanies a periodic recall examination. Radiographic screening of children for malocclusion has not been shown to be of benefit to the community and in general is not recommended.

Filtration
Absorbers or filters (usually aluminium) may be used to remove low-energy (less penetrating) radiation from the beam. These 'soft' X-rays otherwise add to the patient absorbed dose and do not improve the diagnostic image. X-ray machines operating at 70 kilovoltage peak (kVp) or greater usually require total filtration equivalent to 2.5 millimetres of aluminium.

Collimation
This is where a device (e.g. lead disc or metal tube) of varying size and shape is used to restrict the volume of the beam to the

area of interest, thereby minimizing the patient exposure. In intra-oral radiography, converting from circular to rectangular collimation of the beam can reduce the area of irradiated skin significantly (60–70%). In dental panoramic tomography (DPT) accurate collimation of the beam height will avoid any unnecessary irradiation of the eyes and the thyroid. In cephalometry, collimation can be used to restrict the field of view/exposure to the facial bones and cranial base (50% reduction).

Film/screen combination
Intensifying screens are usually utilized in extra-oral radiography. They contain fluorescent phosphorus which emits light when excited by contact with X-rays which means that an adequately exposed film may be obtained for less dosage to the patient. The most commonly used rare-earth screens are approximately five times more sensitive than calcium tungstate screens.

Exposure factors
The kilovoltage peak determines the energy quality (and hence the penetration) of the X-rays. A relatively high kVp (70–90) will keep the patient exposure to a minimum. The milliampere-seconds (mAs) determine the number of photons (quantity) and therefore affect the density of the radiograph.

Film selection
High-speed intra-oral film (E-speed rather than D-speed) should be used to achieve up to 50% reduction in dose.

Lead apron and thyroid collar
A lead apron reduces exposure of the reproductive organs and haematopoietic tissues from scatter radiation. Its routine use is advisable and mandatory in pregnancy. A thyroid collar should be used in cephalometry.

Paediatric radiography
The majority of orthodontic patients are children. Since they are both growing and developing, their tissues are generally at higher risk from radiation. Therefore it is important that radiation protection procedures are rigidly enforced.

Generally, children require smaller radiation doses than adults since their tissues are reduced both in thickness and density. As a consequence, it is often possible to employ a reduced exposure time or a lower milliamperage. Since children have a tendency to move when radiographs are being taken, it is best to decrease the exposure time rather than the milliamperage. This prevents blurring and produces a more consistently sharp image.

Quality assurance programme

The purpose of a quality assurance programme is to produce radiographs that are of high quality with maximum diagnostic information, while using the least amount of radiation. They should also be produced at minimum financial cost. This programme includes processing and dark-room quality control. A radiograph is only as good as the dark-room in which it is developed. The room should be light-proofed with adequate safe-lighting (correct wattage of bulb and correct filter and distance), and all chemicals should be kept fresh while having been prepared and stored to manufacturers' recommendations.

It is estimated that the elimination of clinically unhelpful examinations, in conjunction with a reduction in the numbers of repeat films and the implementation of quality assurance programmes, would result in a 50% reduction of the current collective dose to the population from medical radiography.

During radiographic examinations, sound infection control procedures must be adopted. Examples of this would include wearing gloves, disinfecting areas touched by the operator and placing exposed intra-oral films in a container prior to development.

General orthodontic indications for dental radiographs

Intra- and extra-oral views

The main function of *lateral cephalometric skull films* is to produce a record of the developing face and dentition (see Figure 2.6). The need, use and analysis of such films have been discussed previously in Chapter 2.

For general assessment and when dental panoramic tomography is not available, *right and left lateral oblique or bimolar projections* (Figure 17.1) may be taken, together with *upper and lower central oblique occlusals*. The *bimolar* is an oblique lateral projection designed to show premolars and molars in both jaws on the same radiograph. By careful application of a lead screen to cover half of the cassette at each exposure, it is possible to fit both sides of the jaws on one film.

The *upper central occlusal* is usually taken together with a *dental panoramic tomogram* to search for a supernumerary tooth

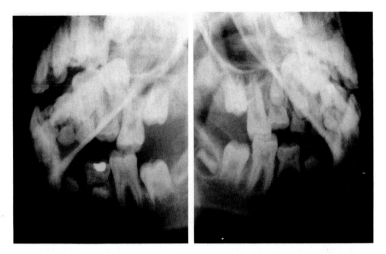

Figure 17.1 Bimolar or lateral oblique radiographs. Note the congenital absence of the maxillary second premolar on the patient's right side (left radiograph) and congenital absence of the mandibular second premolar on the patient's left side (right radiograph). The artefact on the left radiograph below the border of the mandible is a metal stud-fastener on the patient's jacket

or an odontome. A small mesiodens can sometimes be missed on panoramic projections if it lies outside the focal trough.

The *vertex occlusal film* is taken with the X-ray beam aimed down the root of the upper incisors. It gives a plan view of the upper arch and has often been used in the past to localize an unerupted upper canine. However, this projection is not recommended for regular use in contemporary practice, as it gives an unacceptable level of radiation dose for usually poor contrast and detail. On the rare occasions that it proves necessary to employ this view, a dental X-ray set with a capability in excess of 65 kV should be employed, together with an intra-oral cassette containing intensifying screens. A lead apron should protect the gonads.

The panoramic or bimolar projections may need to be supplemented by appropriate *peri-apical films* where additional fine detail might be necessary, as in suspicion of root resorption, dilaceration or other similar dental malformations.

Dental panoramic tomograph

This film is useful when a comprehensive dental examination, including dental development, anomalies and pathology of the jaws, is desirable (Figure 6.2). The temporomandibular joints and maxillary sinuses are also depicted. This projection is relatively easy to perform and has the added value of a reduction of radiation when compared with a series of full-mouth intra-oral films. This latter approach would be rarely indicated in the orthodontic clinic.

It is important to appreciate that the DPT differs from conventional radiographs by being a sectional radiograph, and only the structures within the section (focal trough or zone of sharpness) will be in focus in the final image. The other structures on both sides of the section will be blurred and degrade the picture.

The principles of panoramic imaging are described in specialized textbooks (Whaite, 1992). The discussion here will be confined only to important points, which should be understood as they influence both image quality and interpretation.

Since the DPT has a predetermined focal trough corresponding to the average shape of the dental arch, the distortion and unsharpness of the image increases as the dental arch diverges from the norm. The focal trough narrows anteriorly which means that often even a quite small positioning error of the incisor teeth could greatly distort the local image. Magnification in panoramic radiography is complex because the ratio of the focus–object to the object–film distance is not everywhere identical. Magnification also varies across the film and from patient to patient. In practical terms this means that the size of teeth may be over- or under-estimated and the inclination/angulation of teeth cannot be accurately perceived.

Common artefacts might include ghost images of the hard palate and nasal structures (usually overlapping the maxillary sinus of the opposite side), the mandibular ramus of the other side and cervical vertebrae. Ghost images are the result of the projection of structures that are positioned between the X-ray source and the centre of rotation. They are seen on the opposite side of the film enlarged, distorted and at a higher level from the real shadows.

In order to obtain a diagnostic quality panoramic image free of artefacts and positioning errors, the patient must be prepared (i.e. hair slides, spectacles, nose and/or earrings and studs, and intra-oral appliances removed), positioned in the machine with the mid-sagittal plane perpendicular to the floor, and the Frankfort plane roughly parallel to the floor. The anterior teeth should be centred in the focal trough and the neck should be extended.

Further notes on panoramic radiography
1. Where there is an extreme discrepancy in the facial skeleton (Class II or III) the anterior teeth relationships may make it

impossible to obtain a clear image of the maxillary and mandibular anterior segments simultaneously. In patients with an Angle's Class II Division 1 malocclusion, it might be necessary to lift the face slightly during positioning. In Class II Division 2, it may be advisable for the patient to occlude on a cotton roll during exposure to avoid a vertical overlap of the teeth.

2. In the buccal regions, the maxillary teeth show much more overlap than those in the mandible. The image of the hard palate usually overlaps the unerupted teeth or the developing roots.

3. Evaluation of space. In the developing dentition, accurate space measurement is seriously limited. In general, angular measurements are more reliable in the buccal areas. Usually linear dimensions in the vertical direction are enlarged by a more constant factor, whereas in the horizontal direction this effect is more variable, increasing from the mesial part of the film back to the distal.

4. The DPT is of limited use in the evaluation of patients with jaw and other dental asymmetries.

5. A new generation of panoramic radiographic machines has arrived with the development of the 'Scanora R'. This apparatus incorporates zonography software which permits tomography of the temporomandibular joint or cross-section of the jaw. A current drawback to such equipment is the high cost and its value in the orthodontic context still awaits assessment. Among other developments in this area one might anticipate that equipment for producing digital radiographs may become more widely used in the near future. The eventual intention is to replace film-based technology with computer-based devices that may record and then store the image in a digital form.

The localization of unerupted or misplaced teeth

The basis for the localization technique is a change in positional reference (object and the reference object) that results from altering the central ray projection. The relative object–film distance may provide clues: objects closer to a film appear sharper and of actual size; objects distant to the film appear more blurred and enlarged. One method of location is by the application of two different projections (that are at right angles to each other). Another technique, frequently employed in orthodontics, is the *parallax method*, where one standard projection is taken and then

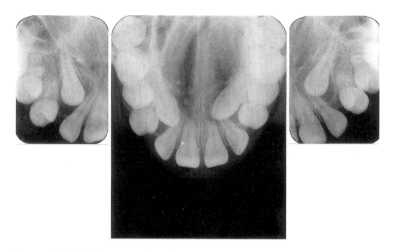

Figure 17.2 Maxillary central occlusal radiograph (centre) with peri-apical radiographs of the right and left maxillary canine regions. Relative to the root of the lateral incisor, on both sides the shadow of the unerupted canine has moved in the same direction as the movement of the X-ray tube. This indicates that the unerupted maxillary canines are palatally placed

the tube shifted either horizontally or vertically with a resultant change in the central ray projection. As an example, a standard occlusal film may be used together with an appropriate peri-apical to locate an unerupted maxillary canine (Figure 17.2). On each film the image of the root of the lateral incisor and the crown of the canine will be visible. The image which moves in the same direction as the X-ray tube is the palatally or lingually placed object. Likewise, the object which moves in the opposite direction to the movement of the tube is buccal or labial. Panoramic radiographs also may assist in tooth location. In the plane of the film, objects that lie in front of the image layer (focal trough) are blurred and reduced in size, whereas those that are behind the image layer appear out of focus and enlarged.

Orthodontic radiographic examinations can be considered in four phases:

1. *Pretreatment phase.* General radiographic assessment as an aid to diagnosis and treatment planning is particularly helpful where extractions and/or apical movements are being considered, and also when local pathology needs to be excluded. A dental panoramic tomograph or alternatively left/right oblique

lateral (bimolar) views, together with the appropriate occlusal radiographs, are often indicated to provide an initial scan of the teeth and jaws in a new patient. True cephalometric lateral skull views are taken to aid orthodontic diagnosis and treatment planning, especially in cases of suspected skeletal discrepancy. Such films may provide a baseline for the monitoring of treatment, provided that they have been properly analysed (see Chapter 2) by tracing or computer digitization.

2. *Monitoring (mid-treatment) phase.* In many cases the more experienced orthodontic clinician requires few monitoring radiographs. However, in more severe cases of malocclusion and/or when two-arch fixed appliances techniques are being applied, lateral cephalometric views may be necessary for periodical assessment of treatment progress (see Chapter 15). Intra-oral radiographs may also be required to assess the progress of unerupted teeth or when root resorption is suspected, evidence of the latter being hypermobility of the teeth or where the root apices are initially blunted, thin or spindly.

3. *End of active treatment phase.* Routine radiographs taken at the end of active treatment do not generally benefit the individual patient. However, there are situations where long-term stability is less certain, due to the treatment itself, aetiological factors or to the unpredictability of future growth. Such cases may require radiographs to provide a baseline from which to assess further changes. Post-treatment films are of most value to a clinician's learning process when they are collected to a set regimen, particularly when constituting part of an accepted research protocol or auditing process. In such situations the taking of films is justified as being of benefit to the population as a whole (National Radiological Protection Board, 1994).

4. *Post-retention phase.* Radiographic examination during the post-retention phase is usually not necessary for the future management of the patient. However, films may be justified in selected cases where there is a clinical indication or as part of the structured learning process mentioned previously.

Chapter 18

Minor oral surgery in relation to orthodontics

Minor surgical procedures can prevent or correct periodontal problems, facilitate and expedite treatment, reduce relapse, add to post-orthodontic stability and improve dental aesthetics for orthodontic patients. It should be remembered that there are anatomical and biological limitations to the distances that teeth can be moved as well as technical problems such as inaccessibility of misplaced teeth. In such situations, carefully planned minor surgical procedures can be of assistance.

A team approach, with discussion of the timing of the operation and alternative approaches to the problem, is essential.

General principles in minor oral surgical procedures

Preoperative considerations

Evaluation of patient. A relevant and thorough medical history should always be taken. This would include conditions which might affect wound healing or susceptibility to infection, and identification of those who require prophylactic antibiotic cover e.g. heart valve defects. It is also important to obtain information on bleeding disorders, allergies and medications which might complicate any planned procedures.

Initially, the proposed procedure should be fully explained to both the child and the parents. This explanation includes an outline of advantages, disadvantages and possible complications, so that the patient or parent/guardian may give informed consent. Anxieties should be alleviated as far as possible and plans made for any premedication that may be necessary. Most soft-tissue and some osseous surgical procedures can be performed on a co-operative patient by means of a local anaesthetic technique. Whether a nerve block or infiltrations are to be used, the discomfort can be minimized by application of a topical anaesthetic, the use of a warmed solution, tissue distraction at the time of needle insertion and avoidance of contact with the periosteum during the slow injection of solution. An aspirating syringe should always be employed to avoid inadvertent intravascular injection which could lead to syncope, toxic reactions or inadequate anaesthesia.

Operative considerations

Asepsis. An aseptic technique is essential in every surgical operation, however minor. When normal tissues are cut and traumatized they become susceptible to organisms from both intra- and extra-oral sources. Peri-oral skin should be cleansed with a suitable solution and the mouth rinsed with an appropriate antiseptic agent. The operator should scrub-up, wear a sterile gown and gloves, use sterile surgical instruments and observe an aseptic technique.

Intra-oral incisions, flap design and suturing. When a mucoperiosteal flap is to be raised, the incision should be made through both layers directly down to bone. The incision is made in the direction of muscle pull wherever possible. In addition, the incisions are planned to avoid cutting major nerves (mental and lingual), blood vessels (anterior palatine, mental and lingual) and salivary gland ducts (parotid and submandibular).

The flap should be large enough to provide good access and visibility while minimizing trauma to the tissues. The base of the flap is usually planned to be wider than its apex in order to maintain an adequate blood supply. The vertical relieving incision is made in the interdental region with the entire papilla included. The incision around the neck of the teeth should be made in the gingival crevice and the integrity of the interdental papillae be maintained. Care must always be taken with the retraction of the flap during the operative procedure.

If necessary, bone can be removed with rongeurs, sharp chisels or burs. When the patient is under a general anaesthetic a chisel is more efficient and less traumatic than a burr to expose a tooth crown or root. It may also be used as a hand instrument under local anaesthetic to 'shave' bone and gently expose a site. At the end of the procedure the wound should be irrigated and cleansed with sterile saline to remove the debris. All sharp bone edges are filed and smoothed, haemostasis being achieved before closure of the wound. The wound margins should be supported by untraumatized bone.

When replacing the flap, the margins should be approximated accurately and should not be overlapped. The corners of the flap are sutured first, starting with the mobile corner to the fixed. The sutures must not be too tight and the knots should be away from the incision to prevent irritation. There should be adequate space between the sutures for drainage to help reduce swelling and the likelihood of any haematoma formation.

Postoperative instructions

These include adequate pain control by proper use of analgesics and/or steroids (e.g. dexamethasone) where appropriate, control of swelling by use of pressure dressings, cryotherapy (ice packs) and topical heat to reduce any swelling that occurs. In addition, prophylactic antibiotics should be prescribed where indicated and adequate fluid together with dietary intake should be maintained. Verbal and written instructions must be provided, drawing particular attention to the need for proper oral hygiene and wound care, together with details of whom to contact in the event of a postoperative complication (e.g. bleeding).

Common minor surgical procedures for orthodontics

Fraenectomy

The maxillary midline fraenum
The presence of a gap (diastema) between the maxillary central incisors may be accompanied by a low attachment of the labial fraenum which, in severe cases, can even merge with the incisive papilla. It has been suggested that if the fraenum is removed, the space may be closed with appliances more easily.

Fraenectomy is an operation designed to remove the entire fraenum and, if necessary, the fibrous tissue lying in the intermaxillary suture between the roots of the central incisor teeth. A fraenectomy may be performed at two main times:

- In the early transitional dentition, when an extremely large diastema (6–8 mm) is present. This procedure facilitates space closure and may prevent ectopic eruption of the lateral incisors and/or canines. On occasion it may lead to some spontaneous space closure without orthodontic therapy, but this is unpredictable.
- In the late transitional dentition, following the complete eruption of the lateral incisors together with the canines and where the diastema has failed to close naturally.

A V-shaped radiographic appearance of the interproximal bone between the maxillary central incisors is a useful diagnostic sign that a fibrous fraenum contributing to the diastema is present; it is also an indicator that it may require removal.

The surgical technique of fraenectomy is described in detail in specialized textbooks (see Bibliography). However, there are a number of points worth stressing. When the two vertical incisions, one on each side of the fraenum, join palatally on the tip of the incisive papilla, the tissue on the mesial aspect of both central incisors should be left. This is very important for the regeneration of the interdental papilla, and gives an improved aesthetic result. It is also important to clear completely all fibrous tissue from the median suture. Following the procedure, a suture is placed high up in the labial sulcus beneath the anterior nasal spine to engage the periosteum. This acts as the anchor suture and helps maintain the depth of the sulcus.

The mandibular midline fraenum
A high fraenal insertion contributes to movement of the marginal gingiva around the lower central incisors when the keratinized tissue has been lost, reduced, detached or where mechanical trauma exists. In these situations, or when a minimal area of attached gingiva or thin tissue are present on the labial aspect of the mandibular anterior region, a free gingival graft is frequently recommended.

The tight lingual fraenum
A tight lingual fraenum with high attachment to the alveolar ridge between the lower central incisors may also contribute to a diastema. This can be divided horizontally near the alveolar ridge, and sutured vertically.

Maxillary canines

The impaction of maxillary canines may occur for a variety of reasons, including crowding and the abnormal developmental position of the tooth germ (see Chapter 6). These teeth have a long path of eruption and during this process may be deflected, most usually palatally. When an upper permanent canine is not palpable in the typical buccal position at 10 years of age, the tooth should be located radiographically and interceptive measures instituted. The progress of the tooth should then be kept under review (see Chapter 6). If the canine has still not erupted at 13 years of age or the patient is first seen at an older age, then further investigations and treatment may be necessary. Not only must the position of the canine tooth be determined accurately by clinical inspection and radiographic localization (see Chapter 17), but the following features should be looked for:

- resorption of incisor roots
- cystic change of the follicle (i.e. enlarged follicle around the crown)
- apical dilaceration
- displacement of related teeth.

A full orthodontic diagnosis, including radiographic assessment and localization, must be made and the chances of eruption either normally or after surgical exposure must be estimated. Possible lines of treatment are as given below.

Leave alone
This may be recommended if the canine is asymptomatic, with no evidence or likelihood of infection, cystic change or resorption of adjacent teeth (e.g. where a horizontal canine is very high within the palate). Regular annual review of these patients is usually necessary.

Surgical exposure
The following criteria must be fulfilled:

- the canine is favourably positioned with its apex close to the correct position
- the potential path of eruption is not obstructed
- there is adequate room available, within the dental arches, to accommodate the canine
- the tooth is not too deeply positioned.

Creating space in the arch prior to uncovering an unerupted tooth is recommended for two reasons:

- if space is not available, the tooth cannot effectively erupt or be positioned in the arch
- the edentulous space in the arch provides an adequate zone of attached gingiva to act as a donor site for an apically or laterally repositioned flap.

The labially located canine. If the eruption of the canine has failed and it is labially positioned, exposure may be necessary. Although the teeth may be palpable labially above the reflection of the mucous membrane, the temptation to make an incision here must be resisted. In order to obtain a sound gingival margin, an 'apically repositioned flap' should be made (Figure 18.1). The gingiva is incised on the alveolar ridge in a semi-lunar shape to

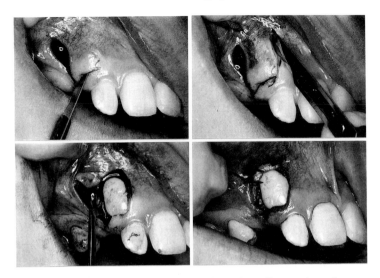

Figure 18.1 Surgical exposure of a labially located maxillary canine using an apically repositioned flap technique. Note how the attached keratinized mucosa has fitted around the neck of the tooth

fit the neck of the tooth to be exposed, and two parallel vertical releasing incisions are made. Once the flap has been freed, the maximum mesiodistal diameter of the crown should be exposed by carefully removing the overlying follicle and bone. Bone should not be removed beyond the amelo–cemental junction. Sutures are placed both mesial and distal to the tooth, to prevent displacement of the donor tissue.

The surgical technique of apically repositioned flap gives a better appearance, while providing a sound gingival margin with an attached, keratinized mucosa which resists inflammation and maintains the depth of the labial sulcus. It has also other added advantages in that dressings are not needed and the dentogingival attachment created helps to prevent marginal bone loss and gingival recession. Following exposure, the tooth will often move spontaneously, although in other cases traction will need to be applied.

The palatally located canine. Where exposure of these teeth is judged to be appropriate (see earlier), the following procedure should be followed (Figure 18.2). After raising a palatal flap to gain access to the palatally impacted canine, the bone over and around the crown should be carefully removed to its greatest

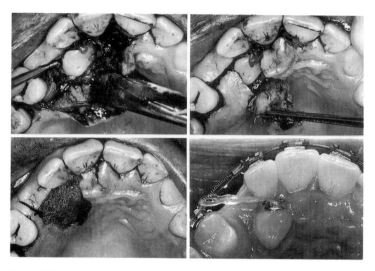

Figure 18.2 Surgical exposure of a palatally located maxillary canine (see text for explanation)

diameter. A channel should then be excised to the alveolar ridge through the palatal soft tissue, taking care to preserve the gingival cuffs of the adjacent teeth. The flap must be sutured back and the opening over the crown packed with a suitable periodontal dressing, for about 7–10 days. The buccal plate and the labial mucoperiosteum should be left intact and the root of the tooth must not be touched.

Where palatal canines are deeper or more poorly positioned they may, after accurate location and exposure, have a gold chain bonded to them. The chain is threaded through to where it is intended that the canine should erupt (on the alveolar ridge) and the soft-tissue flap is replaced. The chain is then attached to a suitable appliance and submucosal traction applied to bring it to a position under the attached gingivae prior to eruption.

Surgical repositioning and auto-transplantation
In carefully selected cases, where there are no medical contraindications, it is possible to undertake surgical repositioning or reimplantation/transplantation of the canine, thereby avoiding the need for either future prosthetic replacement or possibly a prolonged course of orthodontic treatment. The two techniques

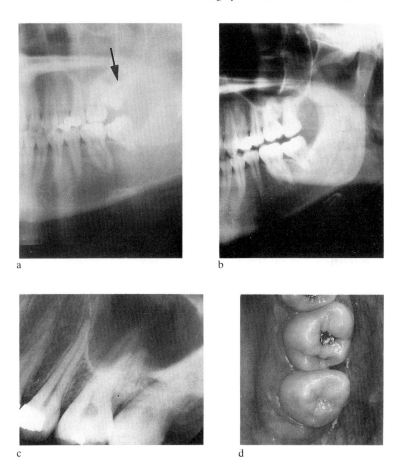

Figure 18.3 Surgical repositioning of an impacted maxillary third molar: a, preoperatively; b, c, three years postoperatively; d, clinical appearance with healthy gingivae

are completely different. The objective of the former is a one-stage repositioning of the tooth, with or without bone removal, into a functionally desirable position, while at the same time maintaining pulp vitality (Figure 18.3). It involves moving the crown in a wide arc around the apex, in an attempt to maintain the blood supply and avoid pulp necrosis. Unlike transplantation the tooth is not removed from its socket. Success in surgical movement of teeth with incompletely formed roots is attributed

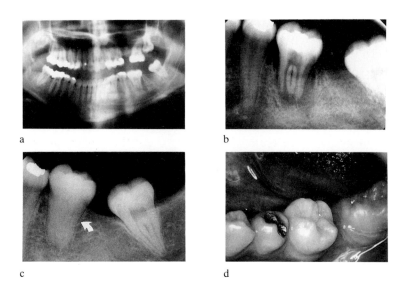

a   b

c   d

Figure 18.4 Autotransplantation of the right mandibular third molar into the lower left first molar socket: a,b, immediate postoperative stage; c,d, two years postoperatively. Note the bone healing around the transplanted tooth with the formation of lamina dura (arrow). Also note the partial pulp obliteration

to the rich vascularity of the apical region and the presence of undifferentiated mesenchymal tissue in the remnant of the dental papilla. This can produce the vascular supply needed in repair of severed or torn tissues. The technique is limited by the availability of space, the degree of root maturation (ideally half to two-thirds of root is formed) and the degree of tooth rotation about the apex that is required. The vitality of the tooth should be evaluated periodically.

Transplantation, on the other hand, is a technique whereby a tooth is reimplanted, after being removed, into a modified or newly created socket (Figure 18.4). As in repositioning, sufficient space must be available (both mesiodistally and vertically) and the rate of success is increased when the root apex is wide open and the socket has been created with minimal trauma. The periodontal ligament and cemental surfaces must not be handled or damaged by excessive manipulation with instruments. Generally, root filling should not be attempted at the time of transplantation but left, should it prove necessary, until the tooth is firm in its new position. It is the contemporary view that transplanted teeth should be root filled with calcium hydroxide during the 3 months following transplantation, in order to minimize the tendency to root resorption. If this procedure is left until signs of resorption are apparent on a radiograph, the long-term prognosis for the transplanted tooth is usually much poorer.

In order to minimize the likelihood of ankylosis, at the time of operation, the repositioned or transplanted tooth should not be rigidly splinted. Partial or total pulp obliteration may occur following either procedure, and root resorption is more common in transplanted teeth, invariably occurring at the cervical margin due to the gripping, with an instrument, of the tooth in this area. Continuing root development is an indication of revascularization and confirmation of a good prognosis. Nevertheless it should be emphasized that transplantation of teeth should only be carried out when orthodontic alignment is clearly contraindicated.

Unerupted incisor teeth

These occasionally require surgical exposure to facilitate their eruption. The criteria are similar to the surgical exposure of labially placed canines. The failure of eruption is often associated with the presence of a supernumerary tooth obstructing the path of eruption of the incisor. In such cases, provided that the timing is right and the position of the incisor is favourable, it will often erupt when the supernumerary tooth is removed. Provided that the incisor is not too high, an apically repositioned flap is appropriate. If, following exposure, the tooth still fails to erupt, then traction may be applied to bring the incisor down into the line of the arch.

Where the incisor is more poorly positioned (as may be the case with a dilacerated incisor resulting from trauma to the deciduous incisors), it is usually very high and not palpable, a gold chain may be bonded in a similar fashion to that described for the maxillary canine. This facilitates submucosal traction to draw the tooth down until it is beneath the attached gingiva, at which time it will either break through on its own or will require a small exposure.

Unerupted central incisors must never be exposed in the non-attached mucosa, since a very poor gingival contour will result and the long-term prognosis for the periodontium is poor.

Mandibular third molars

When fully erupted and correctly positioned, the third molars may form an important part of a normally functioning occlusion. The current view is that these teeth should not be removed unless there is a valid clinical indication. However, impaction is a common problem (see Chapter 7). This may be due to a variety of reasons. One important cause may be the lack of available space due to reduced arch length, something that appears to be increasingly common among the population in modern Western societies. However, even when space is available, an ectopic position of the crypt or an abnormal inclination of the crown may contribute towards the failure of normal eruption and/or impaction.

Currently there is no convincing evidence that impacted lower third molars regularly cause lower incisor imbrication. Therefore, there is no reason that they should be removed routinely for the purpose of preventing later incisor crowding. On occasion however, third molar removal may be justified as part of an active orthodontic treatment plan.

Occasionally, a mildly mesio-angularly impacted third molar may be uprighted orthodontically, usually as part of a simple adjunctive treatment plan.

Early removal
Methods for predicting arch space availability and potential impaction have been advanced and in some studies high accuracy has been reported. However, even in cases where arch length problems are predicted there is little evidence that prophylactic removal of the follicle (by lateral trepanation) or the developing crown of lower third molars is helpful.

Later removal
Unless an impacted third molar is causing symptoms (e.g. recurrent pericoronitis), periodontal pocketing, resorption of the root of the second molar, cyst formation or other associated pathology (e.g. gross caries not amenable to restorative measures), there is rarely an indication for its removal at the end of an active orthodontic treatment. If necessary, the situation of the third molar may be kept under review and a decision regarding its removal made during the latter stages of retention. Generally, third molars are most easily removed when the patient is in the late teens and when the roots are two-thirds formed, although indications for removal are rare at this stage of development.

However, surgical removal of the third molars (particularly in the lower arch) should not be viewed as a routine procedure to be performed on a certain age group as part of the initiation into adulthood. It is a procedure not without inherent risk and complications, and should only be prescribed where there is a definite and current clinical indication.

Supernumerary teeth

Many of the orthodontic aspects associated with supernumerary teeth have already been discussed in Chapter 6. If a supernumerary tooth is symptomless, and deeply buried, it is generally best to leave it *in situ*, but to review its position from time to time. The time interval for review depends on the age of the patient, the depth that the tooth is buried and its recent history (any signs of movement?).

In other cases it is appropriate to arrange removal of a buried supernumerary tooth. This might be indicated if, for example, there are signs of early cyst formation. It would also be appropriate as part of an orthodontic treatment plan if a supernumerary tooth was in the way of any proposed orthodontic tooth movement. If removal is planned, then accurate localization is absolutely essential prior to any surgical procedure (see Figure 6.8, and Chapter 17).

In the majority of cases, remembering the age of the patient and the difficulty of access, these teeth are often best removed under endotracheal general anaesthesia. The surgical approach depends upon their position and the same principles apply as with removal of unerupted canine teeth. It must be stressed that a minimum of bone should be removed to gain access to the supernumerary tooth and that great care should be taken not to damage the standing permanent teeth. Exposure of any unerupted normal incisors and interference with their follicles should generally be avoided since this may lead to the formation of scar tissue, which in itself can impede eruption and so necessitate a later procedure to uncover the incisor.

Fractured roots

Retained roots may interfere with orthodontic tooth movement and it is important that 'routine' extractions are carried out carefully, the roots of the delivered tooth being inspected closely for signs of fracture. Should a fractured root be discovered it is important to extract it with minimal bone removal, preferably by opening a window in the buccal plate (being careful to avoid damage to the roots of adjacent teeth), thereby preserving the height of the alveolus.

Pericision

This procedure is carried out to help minimize the extent of rotational relapse of teeth (see Figure 13.2). Under local infiltration anaesthesia, a no. 15 scalpel blade is passed up the gingival crevice, parallel to the tooth surface, until the blade reaches the alveolar crest of bone. The blade is then passed around the circumference of the tooth thereby severing the periodontal fibres which connect the tooth to the gingival soft tissues. There is no need for sutures or a pack.

Chapter 19

The role of orthognathic surgery

Planning and treatment

The surgical correction of jaw deformity aims to create 'straight jaws', a literal definition of the word 'orthognathic'. Such corrections are largely achieved by osteotomies, a surgical technique by which parts of the jaw are sectioned and then moved into new positions while preserving their blood supply.

Although commonly indicated for moderate to severe skeletal discrepancies of the Class II or Class III type, these procedures also allow the correction of vertical discrepancies (long or short faces), open bite deformities, transverse discrepancies (asymmetries) and congenital craniofacial syndromes (e.g. cleft lip and palate, first arch deformities or the craniosynostoses).

Patient complaints

Patients often present to orthodontists and dental surgeons complaining of the appearance of their teeth. Concerns about their facial appearance and speech are volunteered less frequently, but are often nevertheless present and worrying to the patient. Therefore, a careful history is always important in such cases.

Documentation

Standard records should include:

- a detailed description of the patients' concerns
- facial and dental photographs
- dental study casts usually based in centric occlusion
- an OPT and lateral cephalogram, with a posteroanterior (PA) cephalogram for those patients presenting with an asymmetry
- a detailed dental history and examination
- a detailed medical history and examination.

FRONTAL FACIAL ASSESSMENT

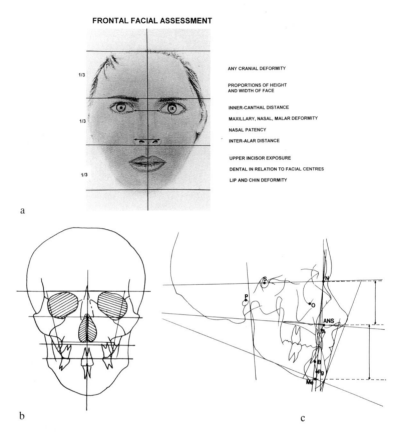

a

b   c

Figure 19.1 a, The frontal clinical assessment. b, The postero-anterior cephalometric assessment. c, The lateral cephalometric assessment

Occasionally, a speech assessment will be required and, in complex syndromes, three-dimensional radiographic techniques (e.g. computed tomography scan reformats) can be valuable.

Analysis

This needs to be based on:

- a detailed clinical assessment of dentofacial form, dimensions and relationships (Figure 19.1a)
- a lateral cephalometric analysis for all anteroposterior and vertical discrepancies (Figure 19.1c)

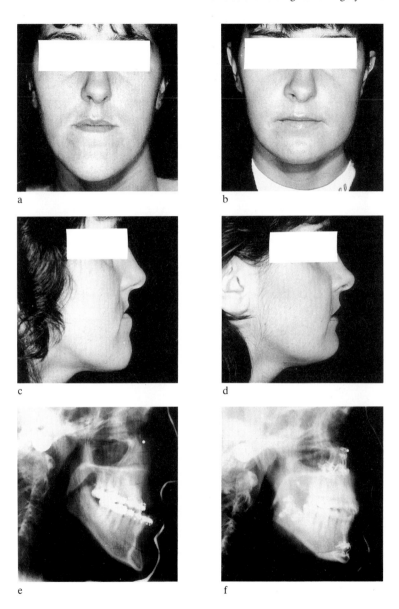

Figure 19.2 a,c, A patient with a Class III (horizontal and vertical) orthognathic problem at presentation: b,d, the appearance of the face after orthodontic and surgical correction; e,f, the surgical change seen on pre- and postsurgical cephalograms

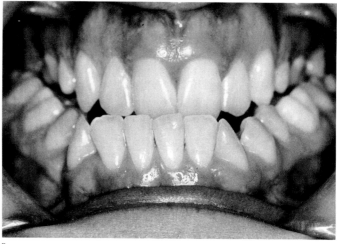

a

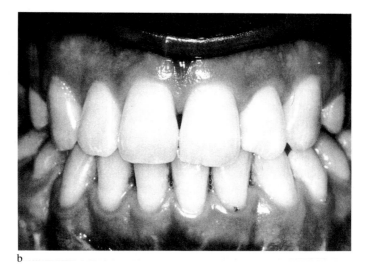

b

Figure 19.3 a,b, Pretreatment occlusion and the occlusal correction
achieved after orthodontics and surgery in same patient as in Figure 19.2
(Orthodontic treatment performed, in this instance, by Mr R. Samuels)

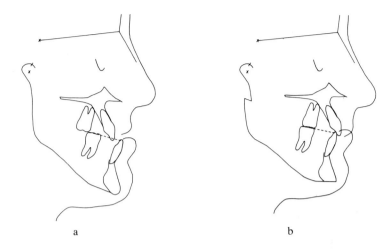

Figure 19.4 a, A computer-generated lateral cephalometric analysis of the patient in Figure 19.2. b, Using the same software (in this instance COG 3.1), a profile prediction tracing, taking into account orthodontic and surgical effects, is generated

- posteroanterior cephalometric analysis for asymmetries (Figure 19.1b)
- a comparison of traced lateral cephalogram films with standard skull templates of the appropriate age and racial group (e.g. Bolton Standards).

By following such a regimen, usually a clear diagnosis can be made. For example, in Figure 19.2 the patient shown has a vertical maxillary excess with an anteroposterior deficiency of the maxilla, anteroposterior excess of the mandible and vertical excess of the chin. In addition, there is significant natural dento-alveolar compensation for the underlying skeletal discrepancy with, in particular, retroclination of lower incisors acting to disguise the underlying mandibular excess (Figure 19.3a).

The presence of any medical conditions or dental problems which may interfere with surgery or orthodontics should be considered at an early stage in the planning.

Presurgical orthodontics

The usual aims of orthodontic treatment prior to surgery are to eliminate any dento-alveolar compensation (and thus reveal the

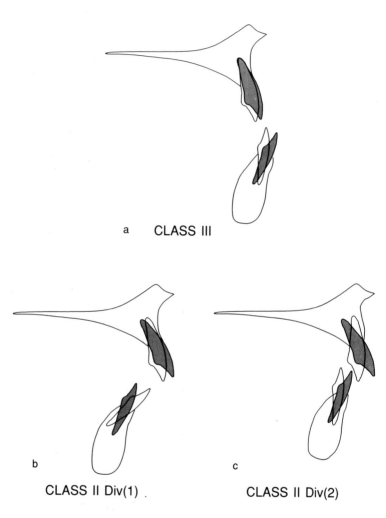

a   CLASS III

b

CLASS II Div(1)

c

CLASS II Div(2)

Figure 19.5 The most commonly presenting incisor position which naturally serves to camouflage the underlying skeletal discrepancy. This is shown for three presenting malocclusions. The shaded teeth show the tooth movements (orthodontic decompensation) achieved prior to surgery

true jaw discrepancy) and create co-ordinated well-aligned dental arches which will be compatible with each other after surgery. This presurgical orthodontic phase facilitates the planned skeletal and facial correction.

In patients presenting with a severe Class III problem the lower incisors are commonly retroclined (Figure 19.5). These pretreatment tooth positions naturally act to 'compensate' and camouflage the original deformity. Presurgical orthodontic correction (see shaded teeth in Figure 19.5) serves to reveal the true jaw discrepancy and thus permits full correction of the facial skeleton by means of the subsequent surgery.

In Class II cases, the dento-alveolar compensation presents typically as shown in Figure 19.5 (Division 1 and Division 2 cases) but often requires similar surgical correction. In all cases, a decision needs to be made on whether the planned orthodontic treatment requires extractions within the arch to facilitate the necessary tooth movements. Such a decision will depend on the need for space and will also be related to the extent of the crowding present. In general, poorly positioned ectopic teeth should be removed.

Once the orthodontic treatment aims have been achieved, large-sized (thick) rectangular arch wires are fitted. Surgical hooks are either fixed to the brackets or the arch wires to aid postsurgical intermaxillary fixation and/or traction.

Planning

Due to the many changes, including those related to growth, that occur during orthodontic preparation, detailed surgical planning will usually be delayed until the last few weeks prior to surgery. It should be based primarily on a sound clinical analysis.

Some form of detailed planning, based on lateral cephalometric tracing principally, is usually appropriate in the attempt to quantify the intended movements of the bones. Such a process may be performed manually by cutting and adjusting multiple tracings. However, this is a tedious process and simple inexpensive computer programs are now available which allow different movements to be rehearsed quickly on-screen. Figure 19.4 shows such an analysis performed for the patient in Figure 19.2. In the average case, such systems can be surprisingly accurate (Eales *et al.*, 1994).

These planned movements are then translated to articulated dental study casts in the laboratory, using reference lines to measure distances. When a maxillary procedure is planned, the models are usually placed on an anatomical semi-adjustable articulator. Occlusal wafers/splints are constructed (in acrylic) in the final and (in bimaxillary surgery cases) intermediate surgical positions to facilitate accurate location of the jaws at the time of operation.

Mid-face surgery

The Le Fort 1 osteotomy (Figure 19.6a)
This is the most versatile, stable and commonly used of all orthognathic procedures. It permits the repositioning of the upper jaw in all dimensions and if necessary the maxilla can be divided into multiple segments. The key to success is to create an ideal position of the upper incisor teeth in relation to the upper lip with their centre line on the facial centre. The anteroposterior discrepancy of the jaws is fully corrected. This will produce an ideal nasolabial angle and a good lip profile. The desired occlusal plane is created by vertical posterior movements and, in anterior open bite cases, posterior intrusion (maxillary rotation) permits full correction.

A sulcus incision from first molar to first molar allows exposure of the entire anterior maxilla which is sectioned with surgical saws and osteotomes along the anterior wall, tuberosity, lateral nasal wall and septum. It is then digitally 'down-fractured' and mobilized with forceps. The bone is pedicled on the soft tissues laterally and palatally. Bony interferences can then be removed, intermaxillary fixation applied across the planned occlusal splint (acrylic wafer) and bone fixation with wires or (more commonly) plates and screws inserted. The postoperative use of inter-maxillary fixation depends on the rigidity of the fixation and personal preference of the surgeon. In the author's experience, it can be avoided in 95% of cases.

Le Fort 2 osteotomies (Figure 19.6b)
These are valuable, especially when there is a genuine anteroposterior (and sometimes vertical) deficiency of the nose and maxilla. When the whole mid-face is involved, including both cheek bones, a *Le Fort 3 osteotomy* (Figure 19.6c) is required. These procedures can sometimes be combined with Le Fort 1 osteotomies in more complex cases.

Pre-maxillary osteotomies (Wassmund, Wunderer or down-fracture techniques)
These are segmental procedures which used to be very popular. Modern fixed band orthodontic treatment ensures that they are now rarely indicated.

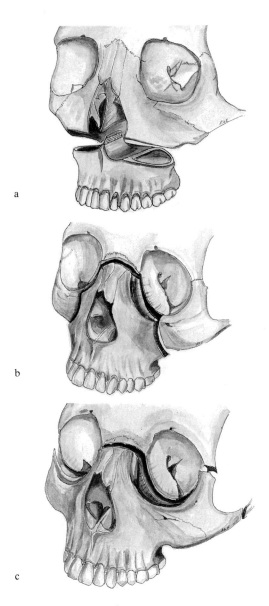

a

b

c

Figure 19.6 The most commonly employed
maxillary oesteotomies: a, Le Fort 1 osteotomy; b,
Le Fort 2 osteotomy; c, Le Fort 3 osteotomy

Mandibular surgery

The sagittal split osteotomy

This is the mandibular equivalent of the Le Fort 1. Although first described by Trauner and Obwegeser in 1957, the modification of Dal Pont (1961) is the procedure most commonly carried out (Figure 19.7a). By splitting the outer part of the ramus from the inner, it permits the entire tooth-bearing part of the mandible to be repositioned anteriorly or posteriorly. It is carried out through an oral approach and can be fixed with screws (often inserted through a small transbuccal skin incision), plates and screws, or wire.

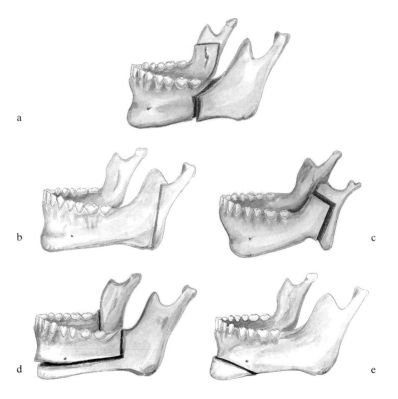

Figure 19.7 The most commonly employed mandibular osteotomies: a, sagittal split osteotomy of mandible; b, sub-sigmoid osteotomy of mandibular ramus; c, inverted L osteotomy of mandibular ramus; d, total sub-apical osteotomy of mandible; e, genioplasty

Its versatility is slightly restricted by the need to avoid length-ening the ramus against masticatory and suprahyoid muscle pull, since this may prove unstable. Advancements tend to be less stable than posterior movements, but there is some evidence that screw fixation and suprahyoid myotomy improve stability in such cases.

Sub-sigmoid osteotomies (Figure 19.7b)
Sub-sigmoid osteotomies of the mandibular ramus were once the most popular technique to correct prognathism and used to be carried out from an extra-oral approach. The procedure can now be performed intra-orally, but it tends to be technically difficult to fix the bones by such a process and may prove less stable than the equivalent sagittal split osteotomy. Inter-maxillary fixation is usually required.

Inverted L osteotomies (Figure 19.7c)
These are indicated when the ramus must be lengthened and advanced (e.g. first arch deformity, condylar hypoplasia). They are usually carried out from an external approach with bone grafts inserted into the spaces created.

Sub-apical osteotomies
These are indicated when only the tooth-bearing part of the mandible needs to be moved. Although usually anterior segments are set up or down, the entire dental arch can be repositioned if desired (total sub-apical osteotomy, Figure 19.7d).

Body osteotomies
These may be valuable in severe prognathism and asymmetry, the cuts usually being made ideally in an edentulous area, interden-tally or after extraction of teeth. The inferior dental nerve is protected.

Genioplasty (Figure 19.7e)
This is probably the most valuable mandibular procedure of all and is normally carried out by means of a horizontal sliding osteotomy. The chin can be advanced in one or two slices, with or without the addition of a bone graft. With appropriate bone removal or grafting the chin can be repositioned in any dimen-sion. Widening and narrowing may also be carried out. This simple operation often produces the most dramatic changes to the profile and overall appearance of the face.

Figures 19.2 and 19.3 show the changes achieved in the Class III case described earlier. Orthodontic decompensation has been

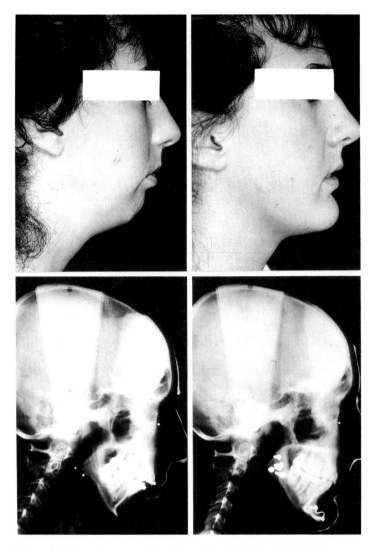

Figure 19.8 A patient presenting with a Class II Division 1 skeletal discrepancy where most of the profile improvement has been achieved by means of an advancement genioplasty

carried out and surgical correction has been by maxillary advancement and intrusion at the Le Fort 1 level, mandibular pushback by sagittal split and vertical chin reduction genioplasty.

Figure 19.8 shows a Class II case where a significant profile improvement has been achieved by means of a relatively small mandibular sagittal split advancement and a large genioplasty advancement. This demonstrates the value of the latter procedure, with a considerable change being obtained in the appearance of the face from this relatively minor procedure.

In almost every case, surgery is followed by a period of orthodontics to finalize tooth position and occlusion. Following the removal of the fixed appliance (debonding), conventional orthodontic retention is necessary. Patients undergoing orthognathic surgery are generally reviewed for a minimum of 2 years after surgery.

Conclusion

Orthognathic surgery is a very worthwhile procedure in suitable cases. However, both the orthodontics and surgery require careful planning. In addition, the overall treatment can take as long as 24 months. Therefore, the patient needs to be highly motivated and the reasons for seeking treatment should be exhaustively explored by the clinicians concerned. Care should be taken to explain the planned changes in facial appearance to the patient. To assist in this process, systems to video-capture images of the face have become available. Such images may then be adjusted by suitable software in order to rehearse the surgery and demonstrate the result to the patient.

Chapter 20

Orthodontic treatment in the adult

The adult patient in comparison to the child

Before discussing the orthodontic options available to this group of patients it would seem worth while to define exactly what we mean by the term adult in the orthodontic context: an adult patient is one in whom growth has ceased to be of relevance in treatment planning for the correction of a malocclusion. For the purposes of the current discussion, this would usually mean a patient older than 16 years of age. This does not mean that there is no growth after this age; indeed, recent evidence would suggest small but significant increments of growth affecting the facial form certainly into the thirties. However, such growth is unlikely to effect any change in the skeletal pattern or soft-tissue profile of the face over the relatively short term of an active treatment. It is also unlikely that such long-term and small increments of growth would be of any assistance in the correction of the malocclusion. For example, both extra-oral traction (headgear) and functional appliances would be of limited use in any adult treatment.

Treatment planning

There is a traditional belief among many clinicians that orthodontic management of the adult is more difficult than that of the child. This is not necessarily true. The treatment need not be any more difficult, provided that it is recognized that treatment planning of these cases needs careful attention, with a number of additional factors needing consideration at the outset.

Past examination of national statistics (Dental Practice Board) would suggest that adult treatments, in general, fail more frequently than those for children, reinforcing the image that orthodontic treatment in this group is more complex. However, such statistics probably more reflect the inappropriate use of simple removable appliances, since in most adult treatments a fixed appliance would constitute the standard contemporary approach.

In fact, there are certain advantages in treating this group of patients, the principal one being the ability of the adult to identify the aesthetic or even the functional problem, these patients usually having a far better perception of their malocclusion than does the child (McKiernan *et al.*, 1992). However, although this type of patient may play a role in deciding treatment goals, it is equally important that their contribution be restricted when it comes to selection of the appliance system. Frequently, it is patient pressure that leads to inappropriate selection of a removable appliance.

Some of the main advantages and disadvantages of treating the adult as opposed to the child patient are listed below.

Advantages

• The facial form and skeletal pattern is largely established. Unfavourable growth during treatment is not a factor.
• The patient is usually able to identify clearly the aesthetic problem.
• This type of patient usually has excellent compliance. There is often an element of self-referral and the patient is strongly internally motivated.
• Since growth is largely complete, orthognathic surgery may be included in any immediate treatment plan where the skeletal or profile discrepancy is to be corrected.

Disadvantages

• No treatment can depend on the assistance of favourable growth. Appliances that depend on such growth for the majority of the correction have only limited use (e.g. headgear or functionals).
• The adult patient is likely to be more demanding when it comes to assessing the final result.
• There can be a problem with social acceptability of fixed appliances for adults in some environments. The improved appearance of the new generation of aesthetic tooth-coloured or clear brackets helps to solve this problem.
• Dento-alveolar camouflage of underlying skeletal problems is only usually appropriate in the milder discrepancies. In the adult patient, greater consideration needs to be given to the effects on the profile of the soft tissues following tooth

movement. This is especially true where overjet reduction is being planned.

- There are often also greater repercussions on the surrounding tissues; for example, ulceration may be a short-term result of fixed appliances, whereas root resorption might be a longer term consequence.
- There is often slower initial movement of the teeth in the adult. Once the turnover of the cells in the periodontal ligament has increased, tooth movement speeds up.
- There is usually more initial pain following an appliance adjustment in the adult. Such discomfort normally recedes after 3–4 days.

There are additional considerations involved in the process of treatment planning the adult:

- having been 'around longer', the adult is more likely to present with retained roots, impactions, apical cysts and other local pathologies
- previous loss of permanent teeth, due to caries for instance, may leave spacing in the dental arch which is poorly placed to assist in the occlusal correction
- there may be areas of significant apical root resorption which could prejudice planned tooth movement
- existing or previous periodontal disease may limit the amount and duration of possible tooth movement
- there may be a history of temporomandibular joint pain which orthodontics could worsen, at least in the short term
- there may be systemic disease present which might affect the treatment approach.

These points, along with others, would need to be addressed prior to commencing any treatment. Any active periodontal disease should be treated and stabilized, while restorations in the teeth should be made sound at the same time that active caries is treated.

In the situation where significant and inappropriate spacing in the dental arches is present, bridgework and/or dental implants may often be a valuable addition to any plan. Conversely, pre-existing bridgework may need to be removed to allow orthodontic correction.

In addition to these general points, careful thought also needs to given to the likely active treatment span: over-ambitious tooth movements should either be restricted or avoided altogether. Decisions on extractions may be dictated by the prognosis of the

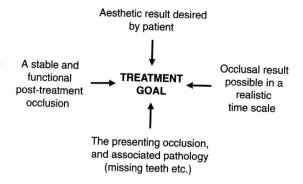

Figure 20.1 Establishing the treatment goal

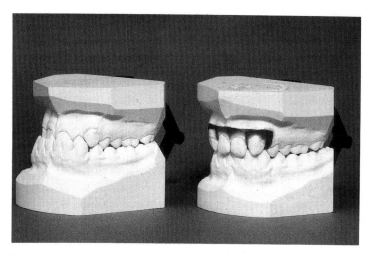

Figure 20.2 A 'set-up' of planned tooth and jaw movements. This is achieved by sectioning then repositioning the study casts

standing teeth; nevertheless some consideration should also be given to the difficulty that can arise in adults when attempting to close excessive extraction space.

In the adult, a perfect occlusal result is not always possible, the treatment goal being determined by a process similar to Figure 20.1. In developing such a treatment goal, the aesthetic correction requested by the patient is an important consideration. The

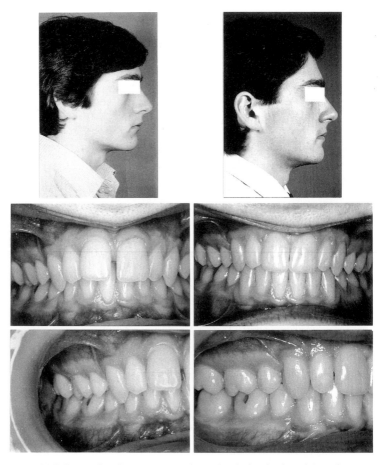

Figure 20.3 Comprehensive treatment of a malocclusion in the adult patient using a preadjusted fixed appliance: (a) start on left, finish on right

patient would also expect this goal to be achieved within a reasonable time scale. As an example, our patients are usually told to expect between 20 and 24 months of active appliance therapy.

The result will also be determined by the presenting pathology (missing teeth, loss of alveolar bone, etc.), but the eventual goal should also be a functioning occlusion – an important factor in the stability of the final result.

In the achievement of a good static and functioning post-treatment occlusion, it must be remembered that post-treatment

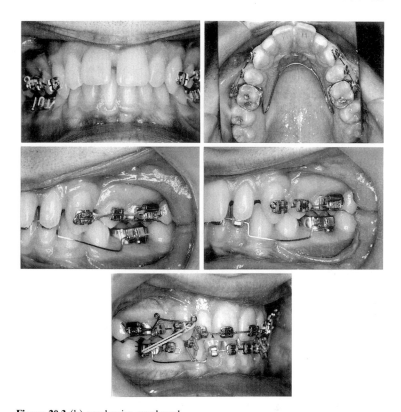

Figure 20.3 (b) mechanics employed

'settling in' cannot be depended upon in the adult as it might be in the child. Therefore the occlusion must be precisely detailed to a conclusion, which is another good reason for using a fixed appliance.

A 'set-up' as shown in Figure 20.2 is often helpful in deciding the eventual occlusal goal, the various options for tooth movement being rehearsed on the study casts.

Treatment

The treatment of adult malocclusion falls into two main categories (Proffit, 1986):

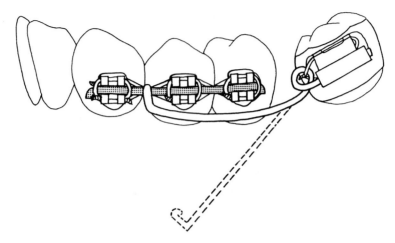

Figure 20.4 Example of an adjunctive type of treatment where a molar is to be uprighted prior to bridgework being placed mesial to it

1. *Comprehensive treatment* – achieving the best functional and aesthetic occlusion possible
   (a) by dento alveolar movements with an orthodontic appliance
   (b) by orthognathic surgery in combination with orthodontic movements.
2. *Adjunctive treatment* – accepting the overall arrangement of the teeth, but making local tooth movements to improve the occlusion while making it both more functional and more physiological. This could involve inter-speciality treatment, for example bridgework.

Comprehensive treatment
This involves full correction of the malocclusion to the best possible aesthetic and functional occlusion. In mild to moderate malocclusions with only a limited skeletal discrepancy this can best be achieved by applying a fully-fixed preadjusted appliance (see Chapter 15) from second molar to second molar to achieve a good dento-alveolar correction (Figures 20.3a and 20.3b). However, since appliances which rely on growth modification (see Chapter 16) are inappropriate in the adult, greater care should be paid to the facial profile, and a combination of

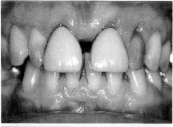

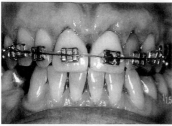

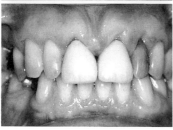

Figure 20.5 Example of an adjunctive treatment where previously periodontally involved and splayed incisors are being brought together, by means of a simple fixed appliance, prior to placement of a splint retainer (Note the enlarged porcelain crowns on the central incisors – this was a previous restorative attempt to reduce the diastema)

orthodontics and surgery will need to be considered in patients with any significant degree of presenting skeletal discrepancy (see Chapter 19).

The treatment time for both dento-alveolar and orthognathic approaches will be similar, as will the appliance which will usually be fixed, with the occasional assistance of an upper removable to allow clearance of occlusal interferences during the early stages of treatment.

Removable appliances as the sole system for comprehensive correction of malocclusion are usually inappropriate in the adult for a number of reasons:

- They are poorly worn due to slow adjustment to speech and eating.
- They do not move teeth with sufficient precision to achieve regularly the desired standard of occlusal finish.

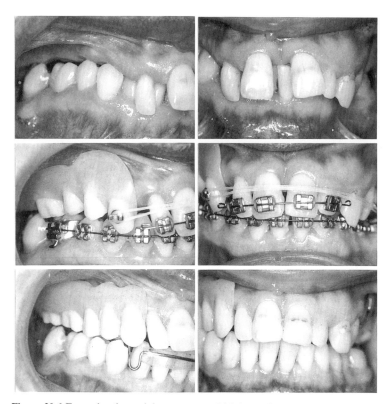

Figure 20.6 Example of an adult treatment which is on the borderline between the adjunctive and comprehensive type. The patient's initial presentation is shown at the top. Numerous teeth are missing and there is a large displacement on closure with a traumatic bite such that a denture cannot comfortably be worn. In addition, the patient is experiencing temporomandibular joint symptoms. In the treatment views note the upper partial denture being used as an anchor while the overjet is being reduced. As a consequence, the incisor spacing (due originally to loss of periodontal support through disease) has been closed. The bottom views show the finished occlusion in retainers prior to the definitive restorative work being commenced

- There is only limited post-treatment settling in such patients.
- They reduce overbite by relative intrusion from an anterior bite plane (see Chapter 14). This is an inappropriate approach in the adult where true intrusion of lower incisors is usually preferred. In any event, bite planes are a much less effective approach in the non-growing adult.

- They are biomechanically less efficient, since ageing changes to the alveolar bone and periodontium will increase the tendency of teeth to tip.

Adjunctive treatment

Where removable appliances may have more of a role is in adjunctive treatments in which limited and usually localized tooth movements are undertaken to achieve a more physiological and functional occlusion. Such treatments are often associated with other dental procedures, for example advanced restorative or periodontal treatments, the aim being to improve the dental health or function without necessarily achieving an ideal or indeed Class I occlusal result which would require the comprehensive approach, previously described.

Figure 15.8 demonstrates a typical adjunctive treatment where a removable appliance has been used to bring a canine crown from its palatal position, eliminating a displacement on closure. Figure 20.4 shows a more conventional treatment where a molar has been uprighted and a plunger cusp mechanism eliminated prior to placement of a crown. Finally Figure 20.5 shows a patient in whom splayed incisors have been collected together following the stabilization of the causative factor (chronic periodontal disease).

Conclusion

Adult orthodontics is a fast-growing area of the speciality. In the USA prior to 1970, this group represented 5% of all orthodontic patients. In the 1980s this was estimated to have risen to between 20% and 25% of treatments. In the 1990s this estimate is likely to be approaching one-third of all orthodontic cases treated. In the UK the trend is probably similar. In a sample of orthodontic referrals to a hospital in Wales in 1985, 26% were found to be over 16 years of age.

When adults are treated, initial tooth movement may be slower and more painful than in the child or adolescent; however, adult patients are generally highly motivated and if planned with expertise may be treated to a finished result of a consistently high standard.

Chapter 21

Orthodontic management of cleft lip and palate

Cleft lip with or without cleft palate is a highly visible congenital deformity of the mouth and face, and is a relatively common condition occurring in approximately 1:700 live births in the Western world. There is some variation in incidence between racial groups. With modern ultrasonic scanning equipment it is usually possible to diagnose facial clefting from about the third month of pregnancy.

Aetiology

The cleft may be part of a syndrome or may occur in isolation. For some there is a clear familial history of facial clefting implying a genetic disorder, but for the majority of cases the occurrence is sporadic, suggesting that as yet unidentified factors have an important role in the aetiology of the condition. Embryologically the nose, lip and primary palate are formed by the fusion of the medial nasal, lateral nasal and maxillary processes in about the eighth week of intra-uterine life. Clefting may arise due to failure of fusion, or fusion followed by partial or total breakdown between the facial processes with continued facial growth. The secondary palate and soft palate fuse in the midline during the ninth and tenth week. Again clefting may be due to failure of fusion or fusion and breakdown.

Pierre Robin syndrome, in which there is a U-shaped cleft of the secondary palate, a retrusive mandible, and a risk of glossoptosis and airway obstruction in severe cases, is thought to arise due to the inability of the tongue to drop down from between the palatal shelves during palatogenesis.

Classification

There is no entirely satisfactory system of classification and this reflects the wide variety of presentation. For the individual patient

224

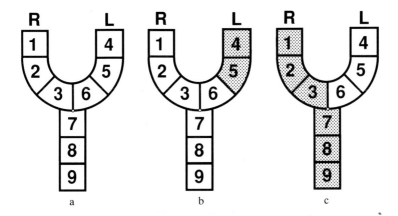

Figure 21.1 a, A simple numerical classification system for clefts – the 'striped Y'. The lip is represented by 1 and 4; the alveolus by 2 and 5; the primary palate by 3 and 6; the hard palate by 7 and 8; and the soft palate by 9. b, Left-sided cleft lip and alveolus only. c, Right-sided complete cleft of lip and palate

it is probably most convenient just to describe the defect. However, for purposes of classification it is useful to divide clefts in three groups:

- clefts of the primary palate: may involve only the lip or the lip and alveolar process as far back as the incisive foramen
- clefts of the secondary palate: may involve the soft palate only or the soft palate and hard palate as far forwards as the incisive foramen
- clefts involving both the primary and secondary palate.

Clefts of the lip and primary palate may be unilateral (most commonly on the left side) or bilateral. In addition, Kernahan (1971) has produced a symbolic method – the 'striped Y' – to describe clefts (Figure 21.1). The small circle at the junction of the Y signifies the incisive foramen. This describes the extent of the cleft by cross-hatching the appropriate squares, and has the added advantage of lending itself to computerized records.

Effects of cleft lip and palate

Dental. The presence of a cleft which disturbs the dental lamina can lead to a variety of dental presentations, principally affecting the maxillary lateral incisor on the cleft side. The lateral incisor may be absent, diminutive, and/or peg shaped with enamel hypoplasia, or it may be of normal morphology. It may appear on the medial or lateral side of the cleft, or there may be a supernumerary or supplemental tooth located in either portion of the alveolar bone adjacent to the cleft. The tooth or teeth will often be displaced palatally and rotated. The central incisor on the affected side will also often be rotated. Both central incisors may have some degree of enamel hypoplasia and this is especially so in bilateral cleft patients. If the central and lateral permanent incisors are displaced, the deciduous incisors may be retained. There is also a delay in dental development on the cleft side, leading to later eruption times.

Occlusal. A Class III incisor relationship is frequently found with a centre-line shift to the cleft side. In bilateral cleft cases, the deciduous dentition may initially be in Class I or Class II Division 1 arrangement, but by the early mixed dentition the effects of limited maxillary growth (see below) are often reflected in a reverse overjet. Unilateral cases will frequently demonstrate a crossbite in the buccal segment, especially on the cleft side, which becomes progressively worse anteriorly. There will usually be a gap in the dental arch in the line of the cleft, as teeth cannot erupt or move into an area with limited bone.

Skeletal. There is often a Class III skeletal relationship, with both the maxilla and to some extent the mandible being retrusive. Until the age of 6–8 years, the bilateral cleft has a protrusive premaxilla. However, with the restraint on growth imposed by the surgical repair early in life there may be change towards Class III (maxillary retrusion) in the early teenage years. There is also an increased anterior face height for both unilateral and bilateral clefts; a lateral open bite may also be found on the cleft side due to a localized failure of alveolar development.

Growth. There is strong circumstantial evidence to suggest that the surgical repair of the lip and palate early in life has a deleterious effect on growth of the facial skeleton, an effect that becomes particularly evident during the prepubertal growth spurt as a developing maxillary retrusion. This is supported by studies of individuals whose clefts have remained unrepaired. In Western countries it is unacceptable to leave a cleft unrepaired, but there is some evidence to suggest that the best results in terms of eventual facial growth come from regional centres where there are just one or two surgeons operating to a set protocol.

Hearing. The muscles of the soft palate act as a valve at the pharyngeal end of the Eustachian tube, equilibrating pressure between the middle ear and the oral cavity and allowing drainage of fluids. Repair of the soft palate cannot always ensure adequate muscle function. Despite early palate repair, suppurative otitis media (glue-ear) is common. This will result in a variable degree of hearing loss, for which consultation with an ENT consultant is mandatory. This may be managed in children by the insertion of grommets (small tubes) through the ear drum, or by the prescription of a hearing aid on a temporary basis.

Speech. Normal speech development depends on good hearing which forms part of a feedback mechanism necessary for the acquisition of correct speech sounds. Inadequate function of the soft palate subsequent to repair may also lead to partial escape of the air stream through the nose, leading to hypernasal speech. This may also occur with a patent oronasal fistula. Other factors which conspire to affect speech in cleft patients are: increased anterior face height, Class III malocclusion, spacing in the line of the cleft, a high-vaulted, narrow palate, and (if a cleft lip was repaired) a 'whistling' deformity of the upper lip. It is small wonder that speech problems rank alongside the dental and facial problems encountered by the patient.

Management and treatment of cleft lip and palate

The objectives of treatment are to allow the patient to: (a) look well, (b) speak well and (c) function well. Ideally this should be achieved by a small team of specialists who treat a high number of cases. Core members of the team should include the orthodontist, oral surgeon, plastic surgeon, speech therapist and ENT surgeon. Contributions to care of clefts from other disciplines are equally important, and omission from the core list does not diminish their role. The general dental practitioner has a vital role in maintaining the deciduous and permanent dentition in a good state of repair and establishing an early regimen of preventive measures: this permits the full range of orthodontic, surgical and restorative procedures to be available for later treatment.

Early treatment
The unexpected birth of a baby with a facial cleft is a considerable psychological blow to the parents, and careful counselling is necessary immediately after birth to reassure parents with regard to the future management and likely outcome of treatment.

Treatment regimens vary both nationally and internationally. Generally, lip repair will be carried out early, within the first 3–6

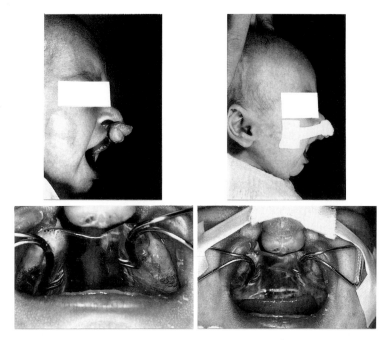

Figure 21.2 A presurgical orthopaedic system being applied in an infant to correct displaced dental segments and soft tissues. This baby has a bilateral cleft of lip and palate

months of life. Surgery may be preceded by a phase of oral orthopaedics to align the displaced cleft segments. This is achieved by the use of an intra-oral plate acting to mould the segments toward each other, and extra-oral strapping working from outside the mouth (Figure 21.2). Such 'plates' carry the additional benefits of obturating the cleft and facilitating feeding, while preventing the tongue from lying between the palatal shelves which arguably might inhibit their growth. They also provide a more normal form to the roof of the mouth which may in turn have benefits for the proprioceptive aspects of speech development. Undoubtedly in some (especially bilateral) cleft treatments, such orthopaedics makes primary surgery a little less difficult (Figure 21.3).

Very early lip repair has been advocated by some who feel that normalization of facial appearance assists parental bonding. The timing for repair of the palate is quite variable, any time between 9 and 18 months being common. Further surgery, in the form of

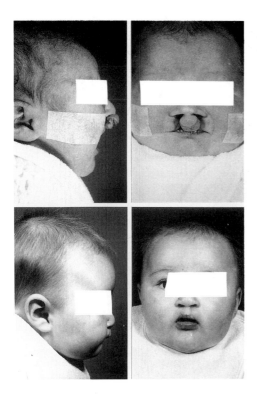

Figure 21.3 The same patient as in Figure 21.2 after 3 months of presurgical orthopaedics (see top right). The lower pictures show the appearance immediately after lip closure (Surgery performed by Mr M. Milling)

soft-tissue revisions to improve the appearance of the lips and nose, may take place in the early years and, for cases with hyper-nasality associated with severe velopharyngeal incompetence, some form of pharyngoplasty may be necessary to help with speech and feeding. This latter type of surgery is intended to improve the posterior seal of the nose and reduce the nasal escape of air during speech.

Regular visits to the family dentist should begin early, with great emphasis being placed on preventive measures.

Early mixed dentition
One or more permanent incisors will frequently erupt into lingual crossbite. At this stage, a simple upper removable appliance may be sufficient to procline the upper incisors to eliminate the crossbite together with the associated anterior displacement. In other cases, a simple fixed appliance might be appropriate. Care should be taken with orthodontic movement where teeth are close to the site of the

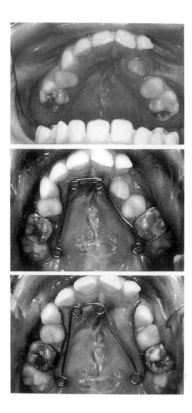

Figure 21.4 A quad-helix appliance being used to expand dental segments prior to secondary bone grafting of a unilateral alveolar cleft (Records by courtesy of Mr R. Samuels)

cleft; in such situations, particularly if an incisor is rotated, it is only too easy to move a tooth out of alveolar bone with an inevitable consequence on the long-term prognosis of that tooth.

Later mixed dentition
Alternatively, correction of incisor crossbites may be delayed until the preparatory stage for autogenous alveolar bone grafting (secondary grafting), which is usually performed at around the age of 9–10 years. Preparation for such a graft may involve expansion of segments comprising the upper dental arch to achieve a normal form. A quad-helix appliance is often used to facilitate these movements (Figure 21.4; see also Chapter 15).

Prior to the eruption of the upper permanent canine, if there is an alveolar defect, cancellous bone is grafted to eliminate the alveolar cleft. The bone is usually obtained from a donor site at

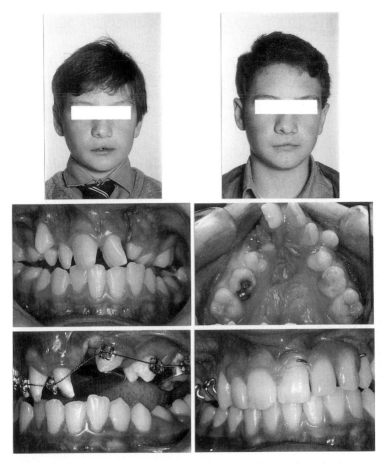

Figure 21.5 An example where correction of the occlusion has been by dento-aveolar movements alone. There has been a secondary bone graft prior to the fixed appliance being placed. A partial denture retainer is in place in the finish picture prior to a long-term restoration being placed. This would be either bridgework or dental implants (Records by courtesy of Mr P. Durning)

the anterior iliac crest. The advantages of this grafting technique are that it stabilizes the maxillary segments, improves the vestibular appearance of the alveolar ridge, assists the closure of any fistula, and facilitates the eruption of the canine into the cleft site. Such treatment also facilitates orthodontic tooth movement and may allow a non-prosthetic rehabilitation of the patient.

Early permanent dentition
Extractions to reduce crowding may be performed at this time as part of a definitive orthodontic treatment plan, the initiation of treatment usually being delayed until the permanent canine has erupted through the graft site (occasionally because of local scar tissue this must be facilitated by means of an apically repositioned flap). Aims of treatment at this stage might include alignment, decrowding, dental centre-line correction and space closure or opening at the cleft site, depending on the case. Full occlusal correction in the early permanent dentition depends on there being no great underlying dental base discrepancy, so that any camouflage necessary can be achieved by dento-alveolar movements alone (Figure 21.5).

The range of orthodontic problems presenting at this stage may vary greatly and therefore a dogmatic regimen cannot be described; thus each case should be carefully examined and treated on its merits. Careful assessment will include an evaluation of the underlying skeletal pattern and the likely effect of any future growth. Where growth is adverse and the patient is developing a significant Class III incisor and skeletal pattern (with an associated poor facial profile), then fixed appliance treatment should be delayed to coincide with any planned orthognathic surgery.

Late permanent dentition (orthognathic surgery)
Once the patient presenting with cleft lip and palate (CLP) enters adulthood they should be reassessed. This provides an opportunity to examine the result of any previous treatments which might include orthodontics, soft- or hard-tissue surgery or speech therapy. Patients in whom large discrepancies of the jaws are developing may be identified. Many may have a significant Class III incisor and skeletal discrepancy with retrusive maxilla such that the middle third of the face will appear flattened or 'dished in'. The patient's concerns, motivations for and expectations from treatment should be carefully explored at this stage.

As in all patients requiring orthognathic surgery, very careful planning is important with, in particular, maxillofacial surgeons working closely with the orthodontist. However, other dental specialities may also need to be involved early in the planning process; for example, the restorative dentist may examine the need for any crown and bridgework as part of the overall plan for the occlusion and long-term stability.

The basic regimen for orthognathic planning is very similar to that described in Chapter 19, as are the requirements for presurgical fixed appliance orthodontics.

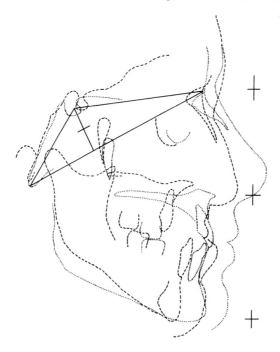

Figure 21.6 Tracing of pretreatment lateral
cephalogram of the patient shown in Figure 21.8,
superimposed on matched outline of a typical non-CLP
patient

Most frequently, a maxillary advancement osteotomy, usually
of the Le Fort 1 type (see Chapter 19), is an appropriate approach
in these patients and very large advancements of up to 2.5 cm are
sometimes indicated. It should be remembered that often the
mandible may appear short in comparison to a normal profile
(Figure 21.6), but it is doubtful whether mandibular advancement
is often necessary. Occasionally, however, if a very large Class III
jaw discrepancy is present a mandibular pushback osteotomy as
well as a maxillary advancement may be necessary to facilitate full
correction of the skeletal and facial profile. In some patients,
movements of the chin (a genioplasty) may prove a valuable
additional surgical procedure in improving the profile of the face.
In the occasional CLP patient, higher level Le Fort surgical procedures are appropriate. These will usually be at Le Fort 2 level,
and sometimes in combination with a Le Fort 1.

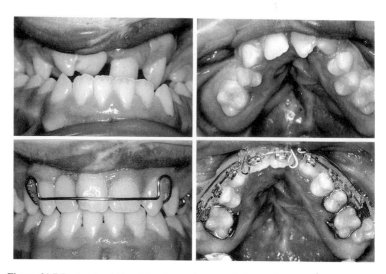

Figure 21.7 Pretreatment/post-treatment intra-oral views of an adult with CLP treated by means of fixed appliance orthodontics, an alveolar bone graft and a maxillary advancement. View on lower left shows occlusion prior to crown and bridgework, but with retainer *in situ* (Surgery was performed by Mr A. Sugar)

In contemporary management of CLP cases requiring orthognathic surgery, the best results are obtained by moving the maxilla forward in one piece following previous alveolar grafting (Figures 21.7 and 21.8). A careful evaluation of the cleft site should be made prior to the presurgical orthodontics, and where there is either a failed secondary graft (or more rarely none at all) the alveolus should be bone grafted at least 6 months prior to definitive jaw surgery. This later procedure is termed tertiary bone grafting.

Retention
Similar to other patients treated by these complex orthodontic and surgical techniques in CLP, all cases should have an individually prescribed system of retention and should be reviewed for a prolonged period of time. Whatever the method of treatment in CLP, stability is notoriously difficult to predict in these cases, due largely to the variable nature of the scar tissue in the region of the repaired cleft, and in many cases some form of long-term fixed retainer may be appropriate.

Some cleft patients, on reaching maturity and when the above treatment is complete, will require late soft-tissue revisions, rhino-

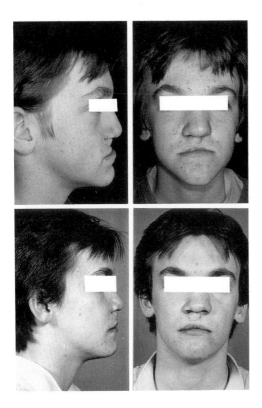

Figure 21.8
Pretreatment/post-
treatment extra-oral
views for the patient in
Figures 21.6 and 21.7

plasty, pharyngoplasty and advanced restorative treatment such as fixed or removable prostheses or implant-retained crowns. Throughout their first 20 years of life, the cleft patient will only derive the best from modern treatment if their dentition is maintained in good condition at all times. The role of the general dental practitioner in this is crucial.

Other craniofacial syndromes

Of course CLP is not the only condition which might affect dental and facial aesthetics and where a combined orthodontic and surgical approach may prove helpful. Other craniofacial syndromes (Treacher-Collins and craniofacial or hemifacial microsomia, Crouzon's, Apert's and Binder's syndromes), although all relatively rare, present at 'combined clinics' from time to time. It is not the place of this text to discuss these conditions in any detail. However, as an example of orthodontics and orthognathic surgery working in tandem in these conditions, the developing facial asymmetry associated with craniofacial or hemifacial microsomia can often be effectively intercepted early in the growth cycle by the combination of a costochondral graft and functional appliance.

Conclusion

This text, for the sake of brevity, has concentrated on the orthodontic and maxillofacial surgical aspects of CLP treatment; it should be remembered that many other specialities are also involved, including restorative and paediatric dentistry, plastic surgery, speech therapy, ENT surgery and audiology, etc. – all should form part of a co-ordinated team. However, in order for these children to obtain maximum benefit from the various treatment regimens described, it is vital that both the parent and child are dentally motivated from an early age and that a high standard of dental care is maintained.

Chapter 22

Occlusal indices

The use of uniform criteria for evaluation of occlusal anomalies is of paramount importance.

An occlusal index may be used to record the various deviant occlusal traits of a malocclusion in either numerical or categorical form. The index may involve direct physical measurement (e.g. overjet), recognition of discrete morphological variations (e.g. crossbite or functional mandibular displacement), or taking the malocclusion as a whole and recording dental attractiveness. Many indices have been developed for specific tasks.

The following criteria must apply to any index:

- it should be clinically reliable and valid
- it should be objective in nature and yield quantitative data which may be analysed
- it should be possible to apply directly to patients or to their dental casts
- it should be acceptable to the profession, third-party payment agencies and the public at large.

Types of indices

Diagnostic classification

These indices are designed to provide a verbal picture of an occlusion to allow communication between personnel. This enables an adequate description of a malocclusion to be made, without the necessity of referring to the patient or the records. The Angle's Classification (Angle, 1899) is the best known example of this type. More recently the British Incisor Classification (British Standard 4492: 1983) has become more popular and is often supported with other information regarding intra- and inter-arch relationships, allowing a full description of the occlusion.

Epidemiological data collection

These indices have been developed to describe the prevalence of various occlusal traits within a population. The epidemiological Registration Malocclusion developed by Bjork *et al.* (1963) is such a system for recording occlusal traits. In a survey of 6398 Swedish schoolchildren (Myrberg and Thilander, 1973) the commonest deviant occlusal traits were as follows:

Crowding	26%
Post-normal occlusion	14%
Anterior crossbite	11%
Posterior crossbite	11%
Overjet greater than 6 mm	8%
Impaction of teeth (excluding third molars)	5%
Pre-normal occlusion	4%

Indices of treatment need

Several indices have been developed to categorize individuals according to urgency and need for treatment. The aims of these indices are:

• to record treatment need in a population and assign priority to cases
• to record health gain resulting from treatment
• to apportion resources including finance, health care workers and facilities.

The Index of Orthodontic Treatment Need (IOTN) attempts to identify and rank malocclusion in terms of the significance of various occlusal traits for an individual's dental health and perceived aesthetic impairment. The intention is to identify those individuals who would receive most benefit from orthodontic treatment. The index incorporates an Aesthetic Component (Figure 22.1) and a Dental Health Component (Figure 22.2; Shaw *et al.*, 1992).

When this index was applied in a survey of 333 Manchester schoolchildren, 33% were recorded as being in need of treatment on dental health grounds and 5% on aesthetic grounds. In a referred sample of 200 patients to a District General Hospital, 74% were recorded as being in need of treatment on dental health grounds and 31% on aesthetic grounds.

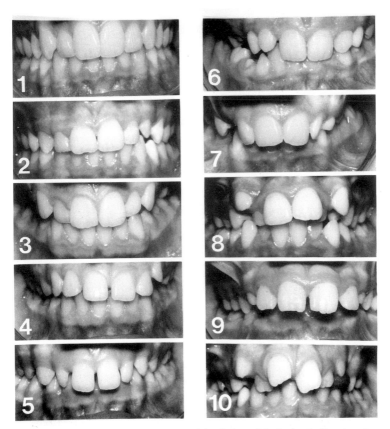

Figure 22.1 The Aesthetic Component of the Index of Orthodontic Treatment Need: the severity of the appearance of the malocclusion is matched to the nearest example and the score (1–10) is recorded

Indices to record treatment standards

These indices compare pre- to post-treatment records to record the outcome of orthodontic care. An index has been developed called the PAR Index (Peer Assessment Rating; Richmond *et al.*, 1991). The PAR Index records the technical quality of care, standard of treatment and the degree of improvement as a result of orthodontic intervention. These indices are useful in determining the efficiency and effectiveness of care both for self-assessment purposes and for comparison of health care delivery systems nationally/internationally. They may also be applied in

GRADE 5 (Need treatment)

5.i Impeded eruption of teeth (except for third
     molars) due to crowding, displacement, the
     presence of supernumerary teeth, retained
     deciduous teeth and any pathological cause.

5.h Extensive hypodontia with restorative
     implications (more than 1 tooth missing in
     any quadrant) requiring pre-restorative
     orthodontics.

5.a Increased overjet greater than 9mm.

5.m Reverse overjet greater than 3.5mm with
     reported masticatory and speech difficulties.

5.p Defects of cleft lip and palate and other
     craniofacial anomalies.

5.s Submerged deciduous teeth.

GRADE 4 (Need treatment)

4.h Less extensive hypodontia requiring
     prerestorative orthodontics or orthodontic
     space closure to obviate the need for a
     prosthesis.

4.a Increased overjet greater than 6mm but less
     than or equal to 9mm.

4.b Reverse overjet greater than 3.5mm with no
     masticatory or speech difficulties.

4.m Reverse overjet greater than 1mm but less
     than 3.5mm with recorded masticatory and
     speech difficulties.

4.c Anterior or posterior crossbites with greater
     than 2mm discrepancy between retruded
     contact position and intercuspal position.

4.l Posterior lingual crossbite with no functional
     occlusal contact in one or both buccalsegments.

4.d Severe contact point displacements greater
     than 4mm.

4.e Extreme lateral or anterior open bites greater
     than 4mm.

4.f Increased and complete overbite with gingival
     or palatal trauma.

4.t Partially erupted teeth, tipped and impacted
     against adjacent teeth.

4.x Presence of supernumerary teeth.

GRADE 3 (Borderline need)

3.a Increased overjet greater than 3.5mm but
     less than or equal to 6mm with
     incompetent lips.

3.b Reverse overjet greater than 1mm but
     less than or equal to 3.5mm.

3.c Anterior or posterior crossbites with
     greater than 1mm but less than or equal
     to 2mm discrepancy between retruded
     contact position and intercuspal position.

3.d Contact point displacements greater
     than 2mm but less than or equal to 4mm.

3.e Lateral or anterior open bite greater
     than 2mm but less than or equal to 4mm.

3.f Deep overbite complete on gingival or
     palatal tissues but no trauma.

GRADE 2 (Little)

2.a Increased overjet greater than 3.5mm
     but less than or equal to 6mm with competent
     lips.

2.b Reverse overjet greater than 0mm but
     less than or equal to 1mm.

2.c Anterior or posterior crossbite with less than
     or equal to 1mm discrepancy between
     retruded contact position and intercuspal
     position.

2.d Contact point displacements greater
     than 1mm but less than or equal to 2mm.

2.e Anterior or posterior openbite greater
     than 1mm but less than or equal to 2mm.

2.f Increased overbite greater than or equal
     3.5mm without gingival contact.

2.g Pre-normal or post-normal occlusions with
     no other anomalies (includes up to half a
     unit discrepancy).

GRADE 1 (None)

1.   Extremely minor malocclusions including
     contact point displacements less than 1mm.

Figure 22.2 The Dental Health Component of the Index of Orthodontic
Treatment Need

the assessment of treatment modalities. A change in PAR score
of greater than 70% indicates a good standard of treatment. In a
survey of treatment standards it has been shown that malocclusions are reduced by 50% in the General Dental Services and

68% in the Hospital Services in England and Wales; this compares to 78% achieved by Norwegian orthodontists.

It has also been shown that upper and lower fixed appliances produce the best standard of treatment.

Conclusion

The use of indices ensures uniform interpretation and application of criteria. It is important before applying indices to ensure that they are valid (i.e. measure what they purport to measure) and reliable (i.e. the ability of the same examiner and different examiners to achieve the same score).

There is a continuous need to improve diagnostic criteria and develop a common approach to assess treatment need, so that those patients who exhibit high priority are treated with the most effective appliances by practitioners competent to carry out the treatment to a high standard. Occlusal indices can be an important aid in achieving this goal.

Bibliography

Adams, C.P. and Kerr, W.J.S. (1990) *The Design and Use of Removable Orthodontic Appliances*, 6th.edn, Butterworth-Heinemann, Oxford

Andrews, F. (1979) The straight wire appliance. *British Journal of Orthodontics*, **6**, 125–143

Angle, E. (1899) Classification of malocclusion. *Dental Cosmos*, **41**, 248–264

Angle, E. (1928) The latest and best in orthodontic mechanisms. *Dental Cosmos*, **70**, 1143–1158

Begg, P.R. and Kesling, P.C. (1977) *Begg Orthodontic Theory and Technique*, 3rd edn, W.B. Saunders, Philadelphia

Bjork, A., Krebs, AA. and Solow, B. (1963) A method for epidemiological registration. *Acta Odontologica Scandinavica*, **22**, 27–41

British Standards Institution (1983) *British Standard 4492:1983*, BSI, London

Clarke, W.J. (1988) The Twin Block technique. *American Journal of Orthodontics*, **93**, 1–18

Dal Pont, G. (1961) Retromolar osteotomy for the correction of prognathism. *Journal of Oral Surgery, Anaesthetics and Hospital Dental Services*, **19**, 42

Eales, E.A., Newton, C., Jones, M.L. and Sugar, A. (1994) The accuracy of computerised prediction of the soft tissue profile: a study of 25 patients treated by means of the Le Fort I osteotomy. *International Journal of Adult Orthodontics and Orthognathic Surgery*, **9**, 141–152

Ferguson, J.W. (1983) A new method of attaching headgear to upper removable appliances. *British Journal of Orthodontics*, **10**, 48–49

Fränkel, R. (1980) A functional approach to orofacial orthopaedics. *British Journal of Orthodontics*, **7**, 41–45

Harvold, E.P. and Vargevick, K. (1971) Morphogenetic response to activator treatment. *American Journal of Orthodontics*, **60**, 478–490

Houston, W.J.B., Stephens, C.D. and Tulley, W.J. (1992) *A Textbook of Orthodontics*, 2nd edn, Butterworth-Heinemann, Oxford

Howe, G.L. (1985) *Minor Oral Surgery*, 3rd edn, Wright, Bristol

Isaacson, K.G., Reed, R.T. and Stephens, C.D. (1990) *Functional Orthodontic Appliances*, Blackwell Scientific, Oxford

Jones, M.L., Nicholson, P.T., and Oliver, R.G. and Robertson, N.R.E. (1992) The place of the bioprogressive technique in postgraduate teaching. *British Journal of Orthodontics*, **19**, 1–13

Kernahan, D.A. (1971) The striped 'Y'. A symbolic classification for cleft lip and palate. *Journal of Plastic and Reconstructive Surgery*, **47**, 469–470

McGuinness, N.J.P., Wilson, A.N., Jones, M.L. and Middleton, J. (1992) A stress analysis of the periodontal ligament under various orthodontic loadings. *European Journal of Orthodontics*, **13**, 231–242

McKiernan, E.X.F., Jones, M.L. and McKiernan, F. (1992) Psychological profiles and motives of adult patients seeking orthodontic treatment. *International Journal of Adult Orthodontics and Orthognathic Surgery*, **3**, 187–198

Myrberg, N. and Thilander, B. (1973) Orthodontic need of treatment of Swedish schoolchildren from objective and subjective aspects. *Scandinavian Journal of Dental Research*, **81**, 81–84

The National Radiological Protection Board (1994) *Guidelines on the Use of Radiographs in Orthodontics* (Report), Northern Centre, Hospital Lane, Cookridge, Leeds LS16 6RW

Oppenheim, A. (1912) Tissue changes, particularly of the bone, incident to tooth movement. *American Journal of Orthodontics*, **3**, 113–132

Oppenheim, A. (1933) Verburgt die Verwendung kontinuerlich wirkender Kraft den optimalsten biologischen und klinischen Erfolg? *Zeitschrift Stomatologie*, **31**, 723–735

Oppenheim, A. (1942) Human tissue response to orthodontic intervention of short and long duration. *American Journal of Orthodontics and Oral Surgery*, **28**, 263–301

Orton, Hs. (1990) *Functional Appliances in Orthodontic Treatment*. Quintessence, London

Proffit, W.R. (1986a) *Contemporary Orthodontics*. C.V. Mosby, St.Louis

Proffit, W.R. (1986b) On the aetiology of malocclusion. *British Journal of Orthodontics*, **13**, 1–11

Reitan (1960) Tissue behaviour during orthodontic tooth movement. *American Journal of Orthodontics*, **46**, 881–900

Richmond, S., Shaw, W.C., Roberts, C.T. and Andrews, M. (1992) The PAR Index: methods to determine outcome of orthodontic treatment in terms of improvement and standards. *European Journal of Orthodontics*, **14**, 180–187

Ricketts, R.M. (1976) Bioprogressive therapy as an answer to orthodontic needs. *American Journal of Orthodontics*, **70**, 241–268, 359–397

Sandstedt, C. (1901) *Nagra bidrag til tandregleringens teori*, Norstedt and Stoner, Stockholm

Sandy, J.R. and Harris, M. (1984) Prostaglandins and tooth movement. *European Journal of Orthodontics*, **6**, 175–182

Schatz, J.P. and Joho, J.P. (1992) *Minor Surgery in Orthodontics*. Quintessence, Chicago

Shaw, W.C., Richmond, S. and O'Brien, K.D. (1991) Indices of orthodontic treatment need and treatment standards. *British Dental Journal*, **170**, 107–112

Trauner, R. and Obwegeser, H.L. (1957) Surgical correction of mandibular prognathism and retrogenia with consideration of genioplasty. *Journal of Oral Surgery*, **10**, 677

Whaite, E. (1992) *Essentials of Dental Radiography and Radiology*, Churchill Livingstone, London

Wilson, A.N., McGuinness, N., Jones, M.L. and Middleton, J. (1991) A finite element study of canine retraction with a palatal spring. *British Journal of Orthodontics*, **18**, 211–218

Orthodontic diagnosis and treatment planning

Treatment planning

1. Introduction and history
Age and sex.
Reason for attendance.
Previous illnesses and accidents.
Habits.
Assessment of interest and co-operation.

2. Soft-tissue morphology and muscle behaviour patterns
Lips
(a) *Morphology:*
  (i)   Competent or incompetent.
  (ii) Habitual position. Whether together or apart.
  (iii) Lip lines: upper, lower and active.
(b) *Behaviour.* The amount of circumoral contraction during speech, expressive behaviour and swallowing.
Tongue
(a) *Size.*
(b) *Position,* e.g. tongue resting forwards between the incisors against the lower lip.
(c) *Swallowing behaviour:* typical or atypical.

3. Skeletal relationships
Assessed clinically and verified from lateral skull radiographs if available.

4. Mandibular position and path of closure
(a) *Mandibular position:* rest or habit posture.
(b) *Interocclusal clearance* or freeway space.
(c) *Path of closure:* hinge movement from rest, or deviation or displacement.

5. Intra-oral examination
Clinical examination aided by models and radiographs.
(a) *General condition of mouth*
Teeth present:
  (i)   Erupted and unerupted.
  (ii) Missing teeth (extracted/developmentally missing).
  (iii) Extra teeth (supernumerary/supplemental).
  (iv) Ectopic teeth and pathological conditions (odontomes, cysts, etc.).

Oral hygiene. Good, average, poor.

Periodontal condition.

Condition of teeth:
  (i)   Caries rate.
  (ii) Damaged teeth/malformed teeth.
  (iiii) Non-vital teeth discoloration; peri-apical involvement.
  (iv) Resorption.

(b) *Tooth positions and relationships*
Upper and lower labial segments:
  (i)   Inclinations and rotations.
  (ii) Crowding/spacing.
  (iii) Relationship – midline; overbite; overjet.
Upper and lower buccal segments:
  (i)   Inclinations and rotations.
  (ii) Crowding/spacing.
  (iii) Relationship – antero-posterior, lateral, vertical.

6. Diagnosis
Summary of salient features elicited in the case assessment (see 1–5 inclusive above).

Treatment plan. This is decided from the diagnosis, a stable final position for the teeth being all important. The co-operation of the patient and parents must also be taken into consideration. Treatment may be: (a) *ideal*; (b) *palliative*.

Practical:
(a) General treatment: conservative, periodontal, etc.
(b) Orthodontic treatment: timing and expected duration, extractions, appliances, retention, prognosis.

Definitions

1. Soft tissues

Competent lips	A lip seal which is maintained with minimal muscular effort when the mandible is in the rest position.
Incompetent lips	When with the mandible in the rest position muscular effort is required to obtain a lip seal.
Anterior oral seal	A seal produced by contact between the lips or between the tongue and lower lip.
Posterior oral seal	A seal between the soft palate and dorsum of the tongue.

2. Teeth and occlusion

Dental arch	The curved contour of the dentition or of the residual ridge.
Occlusion	Any contact between teeth of opposing dental arches, usually referring to contact between the occlusal surfaces.
Ideal occlusion	A theoretical occlusion based on the morphology of the teeth.
Normal occlusion	An occlusion which satisfies the requirements of function and aesthetics but in which there are minor irregularities of individual teeth.
Malocclusion	An occlusion in which there is a malrelationship between the arches in any of the planes of space or in which there are anomalies in tooth position beyond the limits of normal.
Centric occlusion	A position of maximal intercuspation which is a position of centric relation.

Overjet	The relationship between upper and lower incisors in the horizontal plane.
Overbite	The overlap of the lower incisors by the upper incisors in the vertical plane.
Complete overbite	An overbite in which the lower incisors contact either the upper incisors or the palatal mucosa.
Incomplete overbite	An overbite in which the lower incisors contact neither the upper incisors nor the palatal mucosa.
Anterior open bite	The lower incisors are not overlapped in the vertical plane by the upper incisors and do not occlude with them.
Labial segments	The incisor teeth.
Buccal segments	The canine, premolar and molar teeth.
Cingulum plateau	The middle part of the palatal surface of the upper incisor.
Incisor inclination	An expression of the degree of tip in the labiopalatal plane.
Incisor angulation	An expression of the degree of tip in the mesiodistal plane.
Angle's classification	A classification of malocclusion based on the arch relationship in the anteroposterior axis.
Crossbite	A transverse discrepancy in arch relationship. The lower arch is wider than the upper so that the buccal cusps of the lower teeth occlude outside the buccal cusps of the corresponding upper teeth.
Scissors bite	A lingual crossbite of the lower teeth.
Leeway space	The excess space provided when the deciduous canine and molars are replaced by the permanent canine and premolars. The leeway space is slightly greater in the lower arch.
Primate spacing	A naturally occurring space in the deciduous dentition, mesial to the upper canine and distal to the lower canine.
Diastema	A natural spacing between teeth. A median diastema is found between the upper central incisors.
Dens in dente	(dens invaginatus). An enamel-lined invagination sometimes present on the palatal surface of the upper incisors.

Dilaceration	The deformed development of a tooth as a result of disturbance of the relationship between the uncalcified and already calcified portions of a developing tooth. Usually principally affects the root of an incisor.
Microdontia	Abnormally small teeth, often the last of the series.
Oligodontia	The developmental absence of a number of teeth (sometimes incorrectly termed partial anodontia).
Odontome	An abnormal mass of calcified dental tissue.
Supernumerary teeth	Teeth in excess of the usual number – usually of abnormal form.
Supplemental teeth	Supernumerary teeth, resembling the teeth of the normal series.
Buccal segment classification	A classification of anteroposterior malrelationship according to the relationship of the mandibular buccal teeth to the maxillary buccal teeth. The molars are important in this classification but so are the canines (see Chapter 5).
Incisor classification	A classification of the anteroposterior incisor relationship. This is based on the relationship of the lower incisor tip to the cingulum (middle third of the palatal surface) of the upper incisor.

3. Skeletal relationship, mandibular positions and paths of closure

Alveolar process	The parts of the maxilla and mandible the development and presence of which depend on the presence of the teeth.
Skeletal bases	The maxilla and mandible excluding the alveolar processes.
Skeletal pattern	The relationship between the mandible and maxilla in the anteroposterior axis.
Intermaxillary space	The space between the upper and lower skeletal bases when the mandible is in the rest position. It is occupied by the dento-alveolus.
Bimaxillary	Pertaining to both upper and lower jaws.

Prognathism	The projection of the jaws from beneath the cranial base.
Proclination	The labial tipping of incisor teeth often together with supporting dento-alveolus.
Positions of centric	The relationship between the mandible and maxilla when the condyles are in the retruded and unstrained position in the glenoid fossa.
Rest position	The position of the mandible in which the muscles acting on it show minimal activity. Essentially it is determined by the resting lengths of the muscles of mastication and it is a position of centric relation.
Habit posture	A postured position of the mandible habitually maintained either to facilitate the production of an anterior oral seal or for aesthetic reasons.
Interocclusal clearance	The space between the occlusal surfaces of the teeth when the mandible is in the rest position or a position of habitual posture.
Freeway space	The interocclusal clearance when the mandible is in the rest position.
Deviation of the mandible	A sagittal movement of the mandible during closure from a habit posture to a position of centric occlusion.
Displacement of the mandible	A sagittal or lateral displacement of the mandible as a result of a premature contact.
Premature contact	An occlusal contact which occurs during the centric path of closure of the mandible before maximal cuspal occlusion is reached. This may result in either displacement of the mandible or movement of the tooth or both.

4. Cephalometric points and planes

Anterior nasal spine (ANS)	The tip of the anterior nasal spine.
Articulare (Ar)	The projection on a lateral skull radiograph of the posterior outline of the condylar process on to the inferior outline of the cranial base.

Glabella	The most prominent point over the frontal bone.
Gnathion (Gn)	The most anterior inferior point on the bony chin.
Gonion (Go)	The most posterior inferior point at the angle of the mandible.
Menton (Me)	The most inferior point on the bony chin.
Nasion (N)	The most anterior point on the fronto-nasal suture.
Orbitale (Or)	The lowest point on the bony margin of the orbit.
Pogonion (Pog)	The most anterior point on the bony chin.
Point A	The deepest point on the maxillary profile between the anterior nasal spine and the alveolar crest.
Point B	The deepest point on the mandibular profile between the pogonion and the alveolar crest.
Porion (Po)	The uppermost point on the bony external acoustic meatus.
Posterior nasal spine (PNS)	The tip of the posterior nasal spine.
Sella (S)	The mid-point of the sella turcica.
Frankfort plane	The plane through the orbitale and porion. This is meant to approximate the horizontal plane when the head is in the free postural position but this varies appreciably.
Mandibular plane	The plane through the menton and which forms a tangent to the inferior border of the angle of the mandible (or alternatively through the gonion).
Maxillary plane	The plane through the anterior nasal spine and the posterior nasal spine.

5. Radiology terms

Kilovoltage (kV)	The potential difference between the anode and the cathode of an X-ray tube (in an X-ray machine).
Milliampere (mA)	The current flow from the cathode to the anode, which regulates the intensity of radiation emitted by the X-ray tube (milliampere is 1/1000th of an ampere).

Relative biological effectiveness	A factor used to compare the biological effects of absorbed dosages for differing radiation and tissues.
Kilovoltage peak (kVp)	The peak value (in kilovolts) of the potential difference of a pulsating-potential generator.
Exposure factors	Radiographic kilovoltage, milliamperage, exposure time and source-to-film distance. All considered when making an exposure.
Tomography	A special technique which makes the image of a layer of structures more clear than those above and below.
Zonography	A tomographic technique which aims to see the whole of a structure in an undistorted and sharply defined form.
Cosmic rays	Radiation of extremely short wavelengths originating outside the earth's atmosphere.
Background radiation	Implies radioactivity arising from nature (e.g. cosmic rays).
X-ray	A type of electromagnetic radiation characterized by wavelengths of 100 angstroms or less.
Film speed	The amount of exposure to light or X-rays required to give image density. These are classed from A to F.
Localization	The taking of a film to identify a site in relation to surrounding structures.

Appendix III

Standard orthodontic diagnosis form

ORTHODONTIC DIAGNOSIS SHEET

1 PATIENT'S COMPLAINT

Reasons for referral

2 FACE

		Y	N
Asymmetry			
Vertical:	Decreased		
	Average		
	Increased		

Antero-posterior	Skeletal I			
	Skeletal II			
	Skeletal III			
		mild	mod.	sev.

Bimaxillary	Protrusion	
	Retrusion	

3 SOFT TISSUE AT REST

Lips:	Competent	
	Incompetent	
	Competent with	
	mild effort	

Swallow:	Lips closed	
	Lips apart	
	Lip tongue seal	
	Expressive L lip	

Habits

Speech

4 INCISOR RELATIONSHIP

Class I		Overjet	
Class II [1]		(+/- in mm)	
Class II [2]			
Class III			

Overbite:	A.O.B.	
	Reduced	
	Average	
	Increased	
	Complete/mucosa	
	Complete/tooth	
	Traumatic	
	Incomplete	

Centre lines
(to face)

Displacement	None	
to closure	Anterior	
	Posterior	
	Lateral	R	L

5 LABIAL SEGMENTS

Upper		Lower
	Proclined	
	Average	
	Retroclined	
	Crowded	
	Well aligned	
	Spaced	
	Median diastema	
	Gingival recession	
	Fraenum	
	Rotations	
	Cross bite	
	Fracture	

6 CANINE RELATIONSHIP (in units)

	R	L
Class I		
Class II		
Class III		

Angulation:	Mesial
	Upright
	Distal
	Unerupted + palpable
	Palpable buccal
	Palpable palatal

7 MOLAR RELATIONSHIP (in units)

	R	L
Class I		
Class II		
Class III		

8 BUCCAL SEGMENTS

Crowded
Aligned
Spaced
Rotations
Bite

9

Active caries
Teeth poor prognosis
Teeth erupted

10

Oral hygiene:	Good	Fair		Poor

	Y	N
Oral hygiene requires improvement		
Prepared to wear appliance		
Difficulties in attendance		

Anticipated compliance: Good Av. Poor

253

RADIOGRAPHS

U E teeth

Missing teeth

Supernumeries
Impacted teeth

Root resorption

Skeletal classification

I		
II		
III		

Mild   Mod.   Sev.

TRACING

S.N.A. ....   M.M. Angle ....

S.N.B. ....   Interincisal ....
                                angle
A.N.B. ....

Angle to Max. ....

Angle to Mand. ....

To A. Po. ....

L.F.H.

Decreased
Average
Increased

Maxillo-mandibular
planes angle

Decreased
Average
Increased

Bimaxillary

Protrusion
Retrusion

Incisors   Upper   Lower

Proclined
Average
Retroclined

Diagnostic Summary

Treatment Aims

Treatment Plan

Index

255